BORN EARLY

ALSO BY MARY ELLEN AVERY, M.D.

Schaffer's Diseases of the Newborn
(with H. W. Taeusch, Jr.), 5th edition

The Lung and Its Disorders in the Newborn Infant
(with Barry D. Fletcher and Roberta Williams), 4th edition

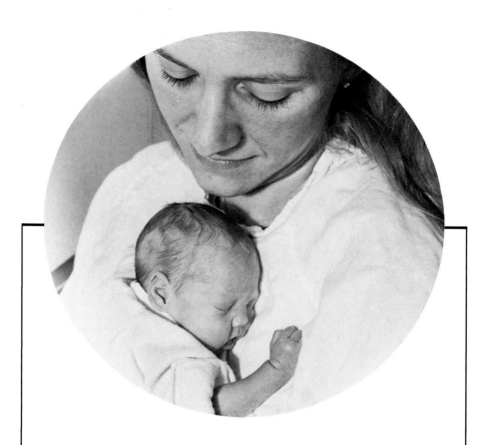

BORN EARLY

Mary Ellen Avery, M.D.
Georgia Litwack

LITTLE, BROWN AND COMPANY
BOSTON — TORONTO

FIRST EDITION

Library of Congress Cataloging in Publication Data

Avery, Mary Ellen.
  Born early.

  Bibliography: p.
  1. Infants (Premature) 2. Weber, Adrienne, 1982–
3. Infants (Premature)—United States—Biography.
I. Litwack, Georgia. II. Title.
RJ250.A87 1983   618.3′97′0924 [B]   83-999
  ISBN 0-316-05865-3

Unless otherwise noted, pictures were taken by Georgia Litwack.

MU

Designed by Janis Capone

Published simultaneously in Canada
by Little, Brown & Company (Canada) Limited

PRINTED IN THE UNITED STATES OF AMERICA

To Adrienne Weber and her family, whose willingness to share their experiences made this book possible.

With acknowledgment to
the Children's Hospital Medical Center
and Beth Israel Hospital
Boston, Massachusetts
and

the more than one hundred individuals who participated in the care of an infant born after 25 weeks of pregnancy on January 29, 1982, with a weight of only 710 grams (1 pound 9 ounces). Adrienne Weber is one of a new group of citizens now given excellent odds of survival and a normal life. We are grateful to all those who cared for her and permitted us to record their efforts on behalf of this infant. In particular we owe special thanks to Drs. Ivan Frantz, Barry Smith, Michael Epstein, and Ann Stark, pediatricians; Drs. Lewis First, Pamela Fischer, Bruce Korff, and Shelly Bernstein, the medical house officers; Susan Shaw, head nurse; Denise Duval, Patricia Rok, and Stephanie Skoolicas, and other staff nurses; Sally Mack, social worker, who also reviewed portions of this manuscript; and Florence Avitabile and John Litwack for their encouragement.

Mary Tondorf-Dick and her colleagues at Little, Brown have been most helpful throughout preparation of this volume.

Preface

I have had the good fortune to witness and participate in the evolution of neonatal intensive care. The environment of the very premature baby, such as Adrienne Weber, has assumed a character that may appear to be one of high technology, automation, and "brave new world," or even "frightening new world," of machines that appear to determine the fate of an individual.

Amidst the advances of medical science and technology I have sensed the exhilarating and ever-rewarding sense of achievement that has been the result of continuing research on the needs of our small patients. But I am also aware of parents' worries and the concerns of individuals caring for the infants, and have wished for more opportunities to discuss the issues.

There is often a communication gap between parents and hospital personnel, in spite of their best intentions. Parents may be reluctant to express their concerns. Physicians and nurses may retreat to the jargon of their professions. Each wants to understand the other, but sometimes the pressure of rapidly changing circumstances prevents leisurely and open communication.

Premature birth brings into focus not only the special needs of the infant but also the concerns of the parents, who are similarly in need of attention. Although many of the kinds of interventions used to support young Adrienne may shortly become dated, the requirements of premature infants will nevertheless always be met by one or another kind of ventilator, incubator, or monitoring equipment. Hardware can change, but neither the babies themselves nor the feelings of their parents are likely to do so.

I was fortunate to recruit the photographer Georgia Litwack to join in this enterprise. She captured the moment, without a single pose, to bring her audience into the intensive care nursery. She witnessed and photographed the drama and the surroundings, and for the first time has documented the changes that occur as a tiny infant grows into a robust baby. The Webers, aware of the value of such a document to other parents, provided unrestricted access and graciously communicated their thoughts and feelings.

We hope, therefore, that some universal and enduring themes will emerge from this journal, and the interventions and the attitudes observed in 1982 will be a faithful chronicle.

For the foreseeable future it is expected that, in the United States alone, 30,000 babies will be born each year weighing under 2 pounds, and another 200,000 will be born with weights of between 2 and 5 pounds. For the parents, relatives, and friends of these infants, we hope that shared experiences as well as clear explanations of the common events that occur in the neonatal intensive care nurseries can provide an understanding of what can appear to be a most confusing circumstance.

The philosopher William James said it best:

"Human nature strained to its utmost yet getting through alive, then turning its back on one success to pursue another more arduous still — this is what inspires us."

MARY ELLEN AVERY, M.D.

Contents

BORN EARLY

BETH ISRAEL HOSPITAL
Boston, Massachusetts 02215

NEWBORN IDENTIFICATION

Parents copy

MOTHER—Name		INFANT—Name		Hospital No.
Weber Frances Sheehan				

Printed Number in Ident-A-Band	Signature, Person Applying Ident-A-Band	Infant's Birth Date		Sex
2419	Rebecca Rosenthron	1/29/82	1:48a	Girl

Signature, Person Taking Prints		Color or Race	Weight	Length
Rebecca Rosenthron			1-9	

INFANT'S LEFT FOOTPRINT
(or palmprint)

INFANT'S RIGHT FOOTPRINT
(or palmprint)

MOTHER'S RIGHT INDEX FINGERPRINT

Signatures, Persons Confirming Sex and Identification

Physician

Delivery Room Nurse

Nursery Nurse

Wayne R. Cohen MD   Rebecca Rosenthron   D... aclyn of Fassde RN

UPON DISCHARGE — Affix Infant's Ident-A-Band® bracelet below and have statement signed and witnessed.

Date_____

I CERTIFY that during the discharge procedure I received my baby, examined it and determined that it was mine. I checked the Ident-A-Band® parts sealed on the baby and on me and found that they were identically numbered _____ and contained correct identifying information.

Signed_____

Witness

Mother

Hospital Representative

Hollister Incorporated, Libertyville, Illinois 60048
Printed in USA.   Form 5815-981

Introduction

Preterm birth is at first a bewildering situation. It is almost always an unexpected event, and there is natural anxiety. What can ensure the infant's well-being in the first days of life? What are the prospects for the future? What is the meaning of all the procedures and machinery that surround the tiny new baby?

This book records the events — sometimes joyous, sometimes alarming, sometimes inspiring — that changed the lives of one young family whose baby arrived unexpectedly after a pregnancy of approximately 25 weeks.

Adrienne Weber was born at 1:00 A.M. on January 29, 1982, with a birth weight of only 710 grams (1 pound 9 ounces). Delivered at the Beth Israel Hospital in Boston, she was transferred within an hour to the neonatal intensive care nursery at the Children's Hospital Medical Center.

Less than 1 percent of all babies are born as early or as small as Adrienne. Birth after 25–26 weeks and before 37 weeks is considered premature. As to weight, less than

2500 grams, or 5 pounds 8 ounces, which usually indicates birth before 37 weeks, ranks as premature, an occurrence affecting about 7 percent of all babies born in this country.

For most women premature onset of labor is unexpected. The symptoms may be subtle at first and resemble gas pains, or menstrual cramps. Persistence of symptoms or an increase in their severity is a reason to consult a doctor. Sometimes a clear vaginal discharge is present if the membranes that surround the fetus rupture. Premature onset of labor is an indication for hospitalization and bed rest. Several kinds of drugs are available that can relax the uterus and stop labor. If labor cannot be stopped, a pediatrician should be notified to stand by and be prepared to resuscitate the baby, if necessary, and mobilize intensive care to provide optimal support for the infant.

The outlook for survival for low birth-weight babies improves each year. Babies born before the advent of neonatal intensive care in the 1960s had few chances of survival if their birth weights were between 500 and 1000 grams (1 pound 2 ounces to 2 pounds 3 ounces). Now more than half of those babies live; the likelihood of survival increases with birth weight. The smallest known survivor, reported in 1973, was an infant born in Poland, weighing only 450 grams (1 pound), who was undersized for the assumed gestational age of 27 weeks. Her weight fell to 360 grams before she began to gain weight. Infants born before 26 weeks of pregnancy with weights less than 600 grams (1 pound 5 ounces) rarely survive. However, with each additional week of gestation, the outlook improves, so that by the time the infant weighs 800 grams (1 pound 12 ounces) or is over 28 weeks gestation, 80 percent survive to be discharged home.

The outlook for normal development has improved for all infants, including those born prematurely. Very small infants continue to have risks for some problems that relate to the reasons for their premature birth, or to the difficulties they may encounter during the precarious days in intensive care. Overall, 90 percent of them will be normal. The remaining 10 percent will for the most part represent the infants who are the smallest or most premature. Some will have major disabilities, such as cerebral palsy or blindness. Some babies will experience lesser disabilities, such as crossed eyes, wheezing, and perhaps some motor incoordinations. Continuing research into the causes of these problems and means of prevention remains a high priority.

When premature birth happens unexpectedly, obviously many questions arise as to what might have precipitated it. Nearly half the time there is no known reason why labor starts prematurely. One factor that can contribute is the mother's age: if she is under sixteen or over thirty-five, the chances of premature birth are considerably heightened. The outlook for the infant is best if the mother is between these ages. Another predictable association with premature labor is the socioeconomic status of the mother. In developing countries, as many as one infant in four may be born with a weight under 5 pounds. In this country, more premature infants are born to mothers from low-income families than to those from affluent ones. The precise reasons for the association are not clear, but contributing events are a shorter time interval between pregnancies, maternal malnutrition, and poor or absent prenatal care. Also, early onset of labor is sometimes induced in an attempted abortion. In all social classes, excessive cigarette smoking is associated with low birth-weight infants. The relationship is seen with one pack of cigarettes a day; smoking more than one pack a day more than doubles the likelihood of a low birth-weight baby. Some of these infants are born early; others may be born at term but are undersized, which is referred to as intrauterine growth retardation, or small for gestational age. The babies' outlook is best if mothers do not smoke at all during pregnancy.

Alcohol can damage the infant before birth, especially if the mother has a consistent daily intake of alcoholic beverages. The fetal alcohol syndrome is the most severe expression of harm that can come from excessive alcohol intake. The infants are undersized for gestational age and may have small heads, as well as heart and kidney malformations. Since there is no known threshold of safe consumption for a given woman, the best advice is abstinence from all alcoholic beverages throughout pregnancy.

Increasingly, the role of previous abortions or miscarriages and their effect on pregnancy is being studied. It is not surprising that there has been research on this issue, since the problem is potentially one of considerable magnitude. Young women who obtain legal abortions are usually unmarried and have had no previous pregnancies. About 65 percent are under twenty-five years of age, and 75 percent are unmarried at the time of the procedure. Approximately one million legal abortions are reported each year in the United States and this figure doubtless understates the true number.

Although there have been experiences reported to the contrary, it appears as if currently, in this country at least, a single previous induced abortion does not on the average affect the outcome of a subsequent pregnancy. Other studies have noted an increase in premature births after two or more first-trimester (first three months) abortions. This risk is greater if abortion occurs after 14 weeks (second, or mid-trimester).

These statistics do not, of course, speak to the problems that an individual woman might have if there were some scarring of the cervical opening or complications associated with the abortion. A dilated cervix is occasionally seen after a previous pregnancy. Sometimes stitches or sutures placed in the cervix make it possible to carry another pregnancy to term. However, most of the time no anatomical explanation is apparent for the modest increase in the likelihood of premature birth after several previous abortions.

Spontaneous miscarriages are another matter, and occur for many different reasons. A woman with a history of infertility or miscarriages has an increased likelihood of a premature infant in a subsequent pregnancy. A given woman's chances of repeat miscarriages can only be estimated by the obstetrician on the basis of the medical findings. However, a single miscarriage in the first trimester is often a random event and may not influence a subsequent pregnancy.

Other events known to be associated with prematurity include maternal infection, which sometimes is "silent" or undetected. For example, a woman may have bacteria in her urine but no symptoms of urinary tract disease. One of the routine tests during pregnancy is an analysis of the urine for signs of infection that might be treated. This is one of many reasons for good prenatal care.

Other maternal problems, such as malformations of the uterus or fibroid tumors, can lead to premature onset of labor. If the mother has cyanotic heart disease (that is, poorly oxygenated blood because of a malformation in her heart), pregnancy may not go to term. High blood pressure, which may occur for the first time during pregnancy, is another condition sometimes requiring early termination of pregnancy.

Multiple births, such as twins or triplets, usually result in babies whose birth weights are lower than a single baby's would be and who frequently are born prematurely as well. They account for about 10 percent of premature births.

Mistaken estimates of the duration of pregnancy may lead to cesarean section a month or two too soon. Such infants may be of borderline prematurity, that is, less than 37 weeks or under 5½ pounds birth weight. However, newer techniques available to obstetricians, such as ultrasound, provide accurate assessment of fetal size and should prevent this type of miscalculation.

Other times, events of pregnancy over which no one has control, such as when the placenta is attached near the cervical opening (placenta praevia) or when it separates prematurely, may precipitate early delivery. Malformed infants as a group are likely to be small at birth as well as born early.

Once a mother has given birth to a premature infant, the risk of premature onset of labor in the next pregnancy is about 25 percent. If she has had two pregnancies end prematurely, the risk of a third premature ending to pregnancy is about 70 percent. The tendency to premature onset of labor, however, is not known to be inherited.

Even when all the known causes of prematurity are taken into account, we are often unable to explain what happened in a given pregnancy. Most of the questions parents ask have no known answer. Mothers and fathers wonder what they did that was wrong. Was it the insect spray, or the vapors from the newly painted bedroom, or the additives in the food they ate? Did frequent intercourse stimulate labor? No known association with any such specific event has been proved. Occasionally mothers will feel that God is punishing them, or they recall Grandmother's admonition that you get what you deserve. Friends may sometimes thoughtlessly inflame guilt feelings by asking, "Why didn't you go to the obstetrician sooner?"

Most parents expect they will have an uneventful pregnancy and a normal baby. Premature labor dashes these expectations, and almost always gives rise to questions about their adequacy as parents. "Why did it happen to me? Now the baby has to suffer for my failure to produce him right," noted one mother who agonized over the number of tests her baby had to "endure." As parents have more opportunity to visit and see their infant sleeping quietly, they overcome their initial fear that the baby "suffers." They make eye contact, and even elicit a smile after a few weeks. In time they realize the infant in intensive care is feeling better and relating to those who care for him or her.

It must be repeated over and over again that having a baby born early is not usually anyone's fault. Most of the time a given cause cannot be found and certainly it is never a penalty for past wrongdoings.

Advances in Treating Premature Birth

In the late nineteenth century and early part of the twentieth, deaths from infectious diseases in the first years of life were so common that it is not surprising to find so few students of premature birth and so few articles concerning the special needs of low birth-weight infants. These small babies were not expected to live. In fact, in the 1940s some authorities thought of birth weights under 3 pounds as incompatible with life, although rare exceptions have always been noted, as in the case of the Dionne quintuplets, each of whom weighed under 3 pounds. Dr. Allan Dafoe, who delivered them on May 28, 1934, wrote, "There were no scales small enough to measure accurately the separate weights of the babies,

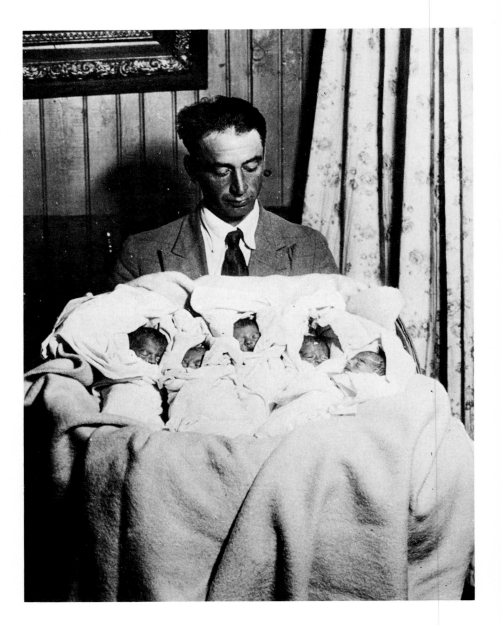

Oliva Dionne holds his quintuplet daughters shortly after their birth on May 28, 1934. (PHOTO COURTESY THE GRANGER COLLECTION.)

but on May 29 (second day) their combined weight was 13 pounds 6 ounces." They were born about two months early. Marie, the smallest, weighed 1½ pounds. Yvonne, the largest, weighed nearly 3 pounds. (Accurate scales arrived on the sixth day!)

As many infectious diseases came under control, physicians turned more attention to newborn babies. As far as we know, Pierre Budin in Paris was one of the first to publish articles on premature infants in 1888. About the same time German physicians, one of whom was Heinrich Finkelstein in Berlin, became interested in the problems of premature infants and initiated special programs for their care. In Helsinki, Arvo Ylppo pioneered in research on pre- and postnatal growth and pathology of prematurity during the period from 1912 on. Julius Hess, an American physician who studied in Europe, was the founder of the first United States premature center at Michael Reese Hospital in Chicago in 1922. The criterion of 2500 grams (5½ pounds) birth weight was used to distinguish a premature from a term infant, and not until much later was the concept of gestational age widely accepted as being more indicative of the stage of development of an infant than weight alone.

Those physicians who were first concerned with premature infants noted very early an inability to maintain body temperature. Various devices, including double-walled metal tubs with the space between the walls filled with circulating hot water, were in use in Europe and Russia in the mid-nineteenth century. Other devices, such as hot-water bottles and electrically heated cribs, were the predecessors of our more modern incubators. Occasionally, the whole room in which many babies were cared for was kept at high temperatures, paving the way for the modern requirements that constant year-round

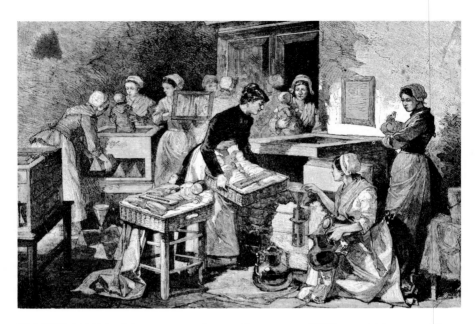

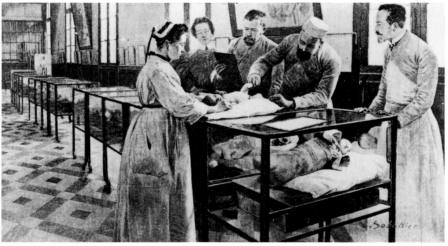

The early incubators used in the Maternity Hospital in Paris were heated with hot water-filled cases; each baby was also warmed by its basket-mate. Dr. Tarnier's incubators (below), introduced in 1884, resulted in the survival of an increasing number of premature infants. (PHOTOS COURTESY THE BETTMAN ARCHIVE.)

temperature and humidity be maintained in the nurseries where premature infants are cared for.

It is not surprising that much attention was focused on ways to feed these immature infants, particularly since some of them were too weak to suckle. Etienne Tarnier in Paris in 1884 is credited with introducing the practice of tube feeding for premature infants at the Maternity Hospital in Paris. Many other devices for oral and nasal feeding of premature infants have been advocated, but not until this past decade has research made total intravenous nutrition possible.

The first physicians to care for premature infants considered human milk indispensable for their welfare. In fact in 1828 Friedrich Meissner in Leipzig, Germany, was so convinced of the benefits of human milk that he advised that the infant be fed mother's milk and be given enemas of milk and at least two milk baths daily!

A number of physicians, puzzled by the inability of many infants to tolerate cow's milk, proceeded to compare the chemical composition of human milk and cow's milk, with the expectation they could modify cow's milk to make it a suitable substitute for mother's milk. In this regard a number of extreme views were taken, including the idea that cow's milk contained an indigestible protein, casein, and that diluting it with three or four parts of water to keep the protein under 1 percent would improve the infant's tolerance to this formula. Later it was felt that a higher percentage of protein was necessary to support adequate growth. In the 1950s the most widely used formula was half-skimmed milk and carbohydrate to increase the protein content and calorie content above that found in human milk.

Over the subsequent years many pediatricians have continued the quest for optimal nutrition for babies of different gestational ages and birth weights, with no universal recommendations. In general, currently, mother's milk is considered optimal, but sometimes not of adequate caloric content, and of course sometimes not available. In those circumstances supplements of easily absorbed sugars and lipids or protein constituents are added to the mother's milk, or modified cow's-milk formulas commercially available are used. The last chapter on the feeding of low birth-weight infants remains to be written.

Some of the early students of premature infants recognized how lethal any epidemics of respiratory tract infection and diarrheal disease could be among such infants. In fact, it was because of the dangers of acquired infection and epidemics within nurseries that special units for care of premature infants were established, to provide separate facilities from other patients who might bring infection to the babies. In the early 1900s the guidelines for care of premature infants specified that incubators that could be easily disinfected should be constructed, that rooms should not be crowded, that personnel should wear gowns and should wash their hands before handling an infant, and that infants with infections should be isolated from others.

It wasn't until after World War II that a new generation of pediatricians focused their attention on the medical needs of premature infants and, working with pathologists, began to study systematically the causes of death after birth (neonatal deaths). Examination of the infants after death showed that not infrequently their lungs were airless, and when examined microscopically revealed a material, hyaline membrane, in the terminal air spaces that should not have been there. From this discovery the condition was named "hyaline membrane disease" and thereafter the label "respiratory distress syndrome" applied to describe the outstanding clinical feature of the disorder. The obvious first assumption was that the material in the lungs was aspirated (breathed in) from the amniotic fluid, but the absence of it in the lungs of infants who were stillborn made that an improbable explanation. Herbert Miller made this point in an article in 1949, suggesting that the affected infants acquired the membranes postnatally. Thereafter many pathologists and pediatricians, through careful study of the infants during their first two or three days of life, and examination of the lungs after death, clarified this condition as a functional immaturity of the lung (see Chapter 3). Because of improved understanding, deaths from hyaline membrane disease have decreased from about 10,000 per year in the United States in the 1950s to about half that number by the late 1970s.

Meanwhile, the 1940s were marked by the construction of many new nurseries and the introduction of more modern incubators that increased the amount of oxygen in the infants' environment. At that time it was evident that some of the infants had a newly recognized eye condition, called retrolental fibroplasia, which by the late 1940s became the leading cause of blindness in this country. The epidemic of this new condition led to enormous speculation about its origin and to a number of studies, which culminated in the work by Norman Ashton in England and Arnall Patz in Washington. When they exposed kittens to high oxygen environments, the kittens acquired the condition. Although oxygen undoubtedly plays a role in retrolental fibroplasia, more recent experience with very immature infants indicates that other as yet undefined circumstances contribute to its severity.

Increased attention to the needs of small babies resulted in a gradual reduction in their mortality. As more very small babies lived, new problems came into focus. Some could be defined for the first time because of the availability of chemical techniques that allowed measurements on very small samples of blood. The application of these newer methods of measurement permitted study of the physiological adaptations of the infant to extrauterine life.

Parallel to increased attention to the babies themselves was the evolution of a field of perinatal physiology, stimulated largely through the work of Sir Joseph Barcroft and his colleagues in England in the 1930s and 1940s, and subsequently by many of their students and colleagues in the 1950s and thereafter. The fetal lamb became the experimental model because the animal could be delivered from the uterus with umbilical cord intact and continue to receive oxygen and remove carbon dioxide across the placenta since the uterus of the ewe does not contract under these circumstances. More recently, it has been possible to place catheters in vessels in the fetal lamb in the uterus for more physiological studies of fetal life. The events surrounding delivery could then be witnessed in a carefully controlled manner with suitable measurements made to define qualitatively and quantitatively changes in the heart and lungs at birth. From these studies many suggestions emerged for less direct measurements on the infants than were possible without jeopardizing their condition.

The 1960s and 1970s were marked by the emergence of a new subspecialty of pediatrics called neonatology. Improved instrumentation and microchemical analyses permitted careful control of the environment of the infants. Pediatricians who have received special training in the care of sick infants, neonatologists, and nurse specialists in neonatal intensive care look after the many needs of the babies.

Neonatal intensive care units exist in almost all major medical centers. Regionalization of care has evolved in most states, so that expectant mothers who are at risk of having infants born early are encouraged to deliver their babies in centers where neonatal intensive care is available. If the baby has problems that were not anticipated, transport to an appropriate center is usually possible, sometimes by air, more often by ambulance. Neonatal intensive care, as we know it in the 1980s, applies the cumulative knowledge of fetal and neonatal life to our small patients, who, although born early, now have a greatly improved (and ever-improving) outlook for normal development.

Many aspects of currently available neonatal intensive care are depicted on the following pages. Ventilators especially designed for premature infants, oxygen measuring devices, and monitors for heart rate and blood pressure are commonly used. What cannot be seen is perhaps most important, the knowledge of the highly specialized and experienced staff who care for these infants. New and effective drugs are available to treat some of the common problems and prevent others. Evaluation of ever more effective drugs through controlled clinical trials becomes a responsibility of those who care for premature infants.

No single advance has had the major effect on increasing the chances of normal survival. Collectively, modern developments have made it possible to welcome a new group of human beings to make their place in history.

1

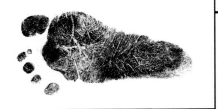

Adrienne's Birth

Franci and Mark Weber, married two years, were anxious to have a baby. In 1981, Franci, a thirty-one-year-old obstetric nurse-practitioner, had lost a baby boy after 20 weeks of pregnancy. She was in excellent health, and the reasons for the miscarriage were unknown. She was encouraged to try again. Mark, also thirty-one, a psychiatric social worker, shared her desire to have a child.

Because of her past history Franci was considered a high-risk patient. Her obstetrician, Dr. Wayne R. Cohen, a perinatologist, examined her frequently. After only 21 weeks of this new pregnancy, her cervix was seen to be thin and judged "incompetent." For that reason the obstetrician placed sutures in the cervix to try to prolong the pregnancy. Franci knew this pregnancy was threatened with early termination, but she hoped she would be able to carry the baby to a point where life was possible even though premature birth was expected. Four weeks later, after premature rupture of the membranes, a small amount of the amniotic fluid that surrounded the baby was drawn from the uterus, examined, and found to have an abnormal number of white blood cells, which indicated the possibility of infection. The decision was made to induce labor even though the baby was still very small and not due to be born for another 15 weeks, on May 12, 1982. The risk of infection to the baby was deemed greater than early delivery.

Franci commented, "I felt I was going to lose this one also and go through what I did last year. Knowing how awful it is to lose a baby made it even harder." She was comforted when she received a full course (4 doses) of the drug dexamethasone, to help accelerate the maturation of the baby's lungs so that it might breathe well even at only 25 weeks of development.

The doctors made preparations for the baby, which included having a pediatrician, Dr. Alvin Faierman, present. Labor was carefully monitored. Dr. Cohen made an incision (episiotomy) to make certain that the baby would not have unneeded pressure on the head during delivery. Franci remarked, "It was such a long shot I didn't expect to have a living baby."

As soon as she was delivered, Franci learned the infant was a girl when the pediatrician said he was taking her to the adjoining treatment room. Franci thought they weren't going to do anything for the baby. "I thought they would come back and tell me the baby died. Meanwhile, I was trying to deliver the placenta and was preoccupied with what was still happening to me. The next thing I knew, another pediatrician, Dr. William Murphy, came to the delivery room and said, 'Congratulations, you have a daughter. She's doing fine. What's her name?'" The Webers had not decided on a name.

The baby did not breathe spontaneously at birth and initially had an Apgar score of only 1. (The Apgar score gives 2 points for each of five important indices of a normal adjustment at birth — heart rate, respiratory effort, muscle tone, reflex responsiveness, and skin color. A perfect score is 10.) By five minutes of age her heart rate had become normal, her color had improved, and her Apgar score rose to 6. A tube was placed in her trachea (windpipe) to permit resuscitation and to make sure she could be ventilated in the days ahead. By the time Dr. Murphy came to see Franci, the infant had been successfully resuscitated and was breathing on her own.

Mark was present during labor and at the delivery and shared the initial grim outlook with some relatives and friends by telephone. He commented he had totally prepared himself for losing her.

Franci was given anesthesia after the delivery since the placenta had to be removed surgically. She next recalls waking in a recovery room just at the time the baby was brought to her. "I wanted to see her but I was pretty much out of it."

Then the baby was taken by ambulance to the intensive care unit at Children's Hospital, a five-minute drive. Mark, who followed by car, commented, "She looked so healthy and active, flailing around grabbing onto her tubes and even crying. She really looked as if she had a lot of life in her. It was hard not to be optimistic, even though we had gone through so many experiences where things had gone from bad to worse."

Franci described the next hours as a state of shock. "I didn't know how I was supposed to feel." As soon as she returned to her room she called her parents to tell them they had a granddaughter at Children's Hospital and she was doing well, but weighed only 1 pound 9 ounces. Still, Franci was encouraged because she knew a baby that size had a chance of surviving.

That afternoon, fourteen hours after delivery, Mark

			APGAR SCORE		
Score	Heart Rate	Respiratory Effort	Muscle Tone	Reflex Irritability*	Color
0	Absent	Absent	Limp	No response	Blue, pale
1	Less than 100	Slow, irregular	Some	Grimace	Body, pink Extremities, blue
2	Over 100	Good cry	Active motion	Cough or sneeze	Completely pink

*Reflex irritability is the response to a catheter in the nostril.

SOURCE: V. Apgar, "A proposal for a new method of evaluation of the newborn infant," *Anesthesia and Analgesia* 32 (1953): 260.

This system of evaluation of the infant is usually carried out at one and five minutes after birth. A score of 10 indicates the infant is in the best possible condition, a total of 7 or more usually indicates a good outlook. Infants who score lower than 7 at five minutes of age deserve continued careful evaluation to find the cause of their depression.

and Franci went to Children's to see the baby. "When we first saw her she had lots of tubes in her. She had an i.v. in her head, and another in her arm. Her chest was covered with leads to measure her heart rate, temperature, and oxygen. I was shocked at how small she was. I had never seen a baby that small," Mark recalled. "One of the striking things is how well proportioned she was. I remember thinking when I saw her hands and features, how adult, how really human she looked. After seeing her we went back to the Beth Israel and stopped by the regular nursery. Those babies looked huge, fat and clumsy. We liked the smaller babies." Franci added, "We saw family resemblances almost immediately. She had Mark's nose and my hands."

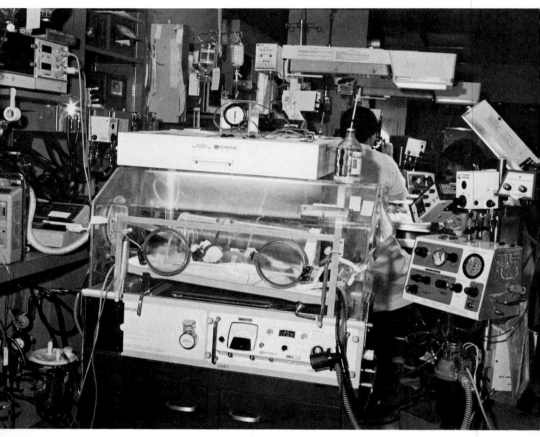

Sometimes it is hard to find the baby in the midst of the hardware! Adrienne is in the center of the picture under a plastic shell (heat shield) to help conserve her body temperature. The incubator is heated to a temperature that will maintain her skin temperature at 36°C. Access is provided by the two circular ports. The white box on top of the incubator contains fluorescent blue and white lights that are used to decrease bilirubin levels by photo-oxidation of the bilirubin. Excessive bilirubin results in jaundice. The large box on the right powers the ventilator and the knobs permit adjustment of pressure and inspiratory time. Another device is the oxygen blender, which adjusts the inspired oxygen to her needs. The box in the upper left corner contains the apparatus to monitor her heart rate and to display Adrienne's electrocardiogram on the oscilloscope screen. Below it is an infusion pump that pushes intravenous nutrients through thin tubes leading to a needle in a vein.

So many wires and tubes! Each one has a purpose. The ones on the chest and abdomen are sensors to detect temperature and oxygen concentration. The wires attached to Adrienne's legs are ECG leads to follow heart rate. The adhesive tape around her mouth anchors the tube from the ventilator, which enters her nose to the trachea. The bandages on the scalp hold a needle in a vein to permit intravenous feedings. (PHOTO BY MARK WEBER.)

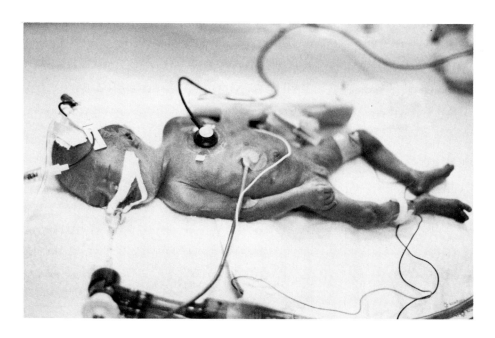

On January 29, 1982, the evening after the baby had been born and transported to Children's, Mark and Franci decided they should think of a name. Mark had been asked her name by the staff at Children's, and he did not want to return without one. They looked through a book of suggested names, and settled on a family name. "Baby girl Weber" was now Adrienne, and it was duly noted on the birth certificate.

Many parents have heard of "bonding" with their newly born infants. Bringing the infant to its mother's arms for fondling and nursing in the minutes after delivery seems a very natural event, one that would have occurred for the infant's protection in the era before the "medicalization" of childbirth. Fathers, now often invited into delivery rooms, may share in holding and stroking their infants.

The resurgence of interest in the immediate postnatal attachment of parents and infant comes in part from consideration of the extensive studies of animal behaviors. A newborn lamb, for example, will "adopt" humans if they become its caretakers and provide milk in the days after birth. The lamb may even remain independent of the flock in its preference for human relationships. A mother goat will relate to any newborn kid for a few hours after delivery, but later rejects any strange kid in preference for her own.

Attachments depend on more than food. In the classic studies of H. F. and M. K. Harlow in the 1950s, infant monkeys had a choice of a comfortable cloth-covered "dummy mother" without a nipple, or a wire screen with a functional nursing bottle. The young monkeys preferred the cloth-covered model monkey from whom they had received no food reward. Later, the Harlows found monkeys raised with dummy models became less caring mothers for their own offspring when compared with monkeys raised by their own mothers. These and other studies have provoked thoughtful interest in our behavior toward our own human infants.

Most of the studies on human infants have focused on healthy newborns born at term (40 weeks). The remarkable ability of these infants to recognize their own mothers' voices within three days of birth, even after limited exposure, astounds most students of neonatal behavior. Even premature infants respond distinctively to their own mothers' voices although not usually as early as three days of age!

Mark and Franci were very anxious to establish early bonding. They knew of the natural childbirth movement, and the studies that suggest the importance of early parent-infant interactions. They were pleased to have been able to touch Adrienne after she was resuscitated and brought back to the delivery room. The needs of such a small infant for special care had to be met in order for her to survive, which was why she was transferred to Children's Hospital, where intensive care was available. Even so, Franci and Mark were encouraged to see and hold Adrienne as often as they could.

Pediatricians usually urge the mother, in particular, to see her premature infant soon after birth. It helps minimize fantasies about the baby's appearance. Anxiety at this point is normal, as is disappointment in not being able to carry the baby to term. Facing reality can be reassuring and give the mother a sense of continuing relationship with the baby. Enforced separation or total delegation of caretaking to a hospital staff imposes an added sense of personal inadequacy on a mother already under stress because of the premature birth.

Doctors and nurses encourage as much conversation with parents as may be needed to share explanations of

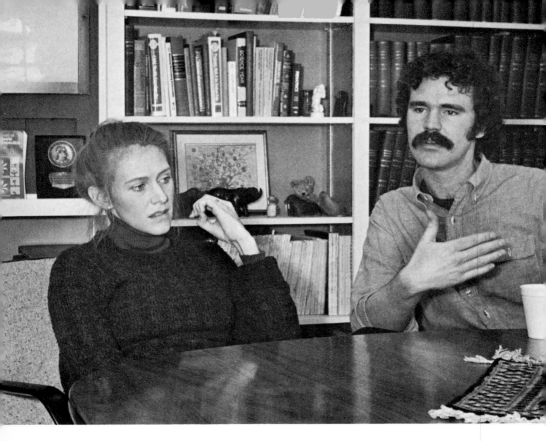

After Adrienne is settled into her new environment Franci and Mark meet with the doctor, to ask about Adrienne's condition and to share their feelings about the past eventful weeks.

the many procedures and the changes in the infant's condition. Sometimes these conversations have to be deferred until the infant is stabilized. Some hours of physical separation from parents may be inevitable if the baby's well-being requires the skill of the team experienced in applying resuscitation, mechanical ventilation, intravenous fluids, antibiotics, and other life-saving measures.

When physical separation from parents occurs, for whatever reason, inevitable or irreversible adverse changes in parent-child relationships do not necessarily occur. Indeed, a wealth of human experience testifies to the possibility of normal and lasting bonding occurring after the first days of life. A baby is not separated from parents by anyone's choice, but by necessity. Surely, parents' involvement with their infant in the hours and days after birth is ideal. A host of circumstances, such as transport of the infant to a neonatal intensive care unit, distance from home to hospital, the needs of siblings at home, and the needs of the parents themselves, are also important in the stressful days after premature birth. For instance, parents with several small children at home might become exhausted if they both tried to visit every day. Parents must find a way to do what they find most rewarding, and trust and share with the professional staff the responsibility of caring for the new baby.

Franci had her own emotional responses to contend with. She recalled that when she was discharged from the hospital Adrienne was only two days old, and "It was probably the most awful day I could remember. I got in the car and immediately started crying. Before then, I kept feeling when things weren't going right, I had to hold myself together. When I got out of the hospital everything started to hit me.

"On the way home Mark took me to a restaurant for dinner. I couldn't stop crying. I must have used twenty napkins! I guess it was a release of everything I had felt when I thought the baby was going to die, then she didn't, but she still might. It was so awful."

Mark had different responses, partly, he felt, because their experiences had been so different. "It's hard to explain," he said, "but premature birth had one positive aspect for me. It was a chance to get to know Adrienne for the first time. All of a sudden, here's my daughter." Franci agreed that Mark was much more positive that things would be all right, and she was more scared. "Mark felt Adrienne was more available to him while I had the feeling she was much less available to me because I was used to having her there all the time. To have her live, then possibly to lose her would be much harder than if she hadn't lived at all, because she was so real to us."

Franci recalled, "You know, it's hard for me to tell whether the amount of worry that I had was based solely on how Adrienne was doing, or whether it was just based on this having been my second pregnancy. Once things go wrong, it is harder to be optimistic than if things had never gone wrong. The first days were the hardest because we had been told if the baby is going to die it would probably happen then. You hang on to every blood test, everything that happens to the baby." Mark added, "You want information, no matter what kind of information. You know that you shouldn't pin your hopes on whether she gains or loses weight, whether her blood gases are exactly what you want them to be, but you want to find out something."

The Webers were surprised and at first concerned by the relative youth of the doctors and nurses who were making so many critical decisions on Adrienne's behalf. The resident doctors are indeed in their twenties, as are many of the nurses. The attending neonatologist, who was senior to the residents, was in the nursery most of the day. When Franci realized that, she felt better. "I quickly got the sense that decisions were being made not by one doctor but by a group of people with a lot of experience, so I didn't worry as much as time went on."

Each baby is assigned a primary doctor and nurse. The parents are encouraged to ask questions of these individuals who are most attentive to the moment-to-moment changes. An attending neonatologist is always on call. Obviously, changing shifts of doctors and nurses require careful "sign out" to provide continuity of care.

One of the reasons for the extensive record-keeping is to keep everyone up to date in an ever-changing situation.

Most parents stay close to their own baby, but even so they sometimes talk to other parents and know the crises in the lives of other families. "Two babies died while we were there," Mark said. "You know, it's difficult to see babies that are sick. One baby across from Adrienne was very sick and it was hard the next day to walk in and all of a sudden see an empty crib, knowing what had happened. We tried to stay away from that as much as possible and not get too involved in what else was going on."

The Webers did not send out birth announcements. They were aware of the uncertainties ahead and the difficulties they would experience sharing these uncertainties with friends.

Given the unnatural aspects of premature birth, it is not surprising that both the infant and parents need time to get acquainted and respond to each other's behavior. Some parents are frightened by their baby's fragile appearance and great sensitivity to stimuli: the rapidity of color changes from pink to gray, the tremulousness, and the irregular breathing that characterize immature responses. Swaddling or wrapping the infant greatly decreases these responses and allows her to relax more. As the infant matures, she assumes a greater capacity to organize or modulate her responses, stays alert for longer intervals, and seems to interact more with parents. These responses occur even before the expected birth date in very immature infants. The timing of this behavioral maturation depends, of course, on the physical condition of the infant and probably on the sensitivity of parents and staff to the infant's needs.

2

First Days

The first week of life is critical for all very small infants. During this period the baby must adjust to being born before all its organ systems have had time to mature. The baby's vital signs (temperature, pulse, blood pressure, and respirations) must be very closely watched. The temperature of the incubator is regulated to within one half a degree centigrade as changes in body temperature dictate. Intravenous catheters supply fluid and nutritional needs, and the amounts are monitored by measurements on small samples of blood. These are just some of the components of neonatal intensive care.

Mark and Franci, who lived only two miles from the hospital, were able to visit Adrienne daily, and daily they shared in some of the concerns of the staff about her special needs. The first day the doctor said the baby had a 25 percent chance of survival. The next day, when she was doing well, they heard the odds were 50–50. Franci began to ask about every test and noted later, "It's like you're hanging on everything that happens to the baby.

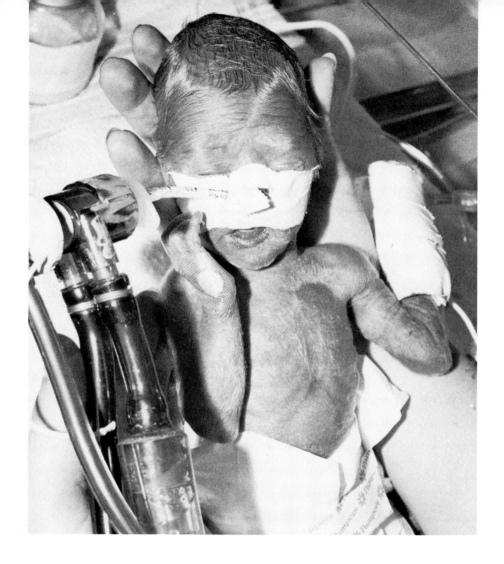

Adrienne is 5 days old. Note the light, very fine hairs on the skin. These hairs, called lanugo, are more prominent in premature infants, but also are present in babies born at term. They disappear after a few weeks. The skin appears wrinkled. At birth, the skin has a higher water content and a gelatinous consistency. In the days after birth it becomes drier. Sometimes skin lotion is needed to keep the skin from irritation. The sparse amount of fat under the skin (subcutaneous fat) makes it wrinkle until such time as the infant begins to gain weight. Outer layers of the skin may even peel, as is evident on her forearm. The bandage on her hand protects the site of an intravenous feeding line. (PHOTO BY MARK WEBER.)

We were told not to follow the numbers, but we could not help wanting to know about the blood tests. We wanted information, no matter what kind of information. When the baby was a week old they were going to start feeding her by mouth and I was feeling very positive. You pin a lot on feeding because that's the baby's ticket out of there. I had been pumping my breasts, and the idea of giving her my milk was very important to me."

Meanwhile Adrienne had shown her first ominous sign, a mild swelling of her abdomen, and a trace of blood in her stools. X-ray films showed signs of a problem with her intestines called necrotizing enterocolitis, or NEC for short. It is a potentially serious problem in premature infants that can lead to a perforated bowel and peritonitis. That meant "nothing by mouth" until the problem resolved. Franci went from a high to a crashing low again. "We didn't know what was going on. One doctor would say one thing, and another disagreed." Although the films were not definitive, the possibility of a potentially serious problem dictated caution. Fortunately for Adrienne, the episode was mild and lasted only two days.

Franci shared some feelings that are almost universal among parents in those critical weeks. "We had a tremendous amount of faith in the staff, which we really needed because we were feeling so out of control. But we eventually reached a point where we sort of fell apart when we realized they could make mistakes. It was very difficult. For example, why was she getting X-rays twice a day when we know you don't ever X-ray a baby in the uterus at twenty-five weeks of pregnancy?" When Franci asked this question, she was told the dose of radiation was very low and the distended abdomen could lead to a more serious rupture of the bowel that could be seen only by X-ray. She had to trust the doctors, but she worried about so much stress for such a small baby.

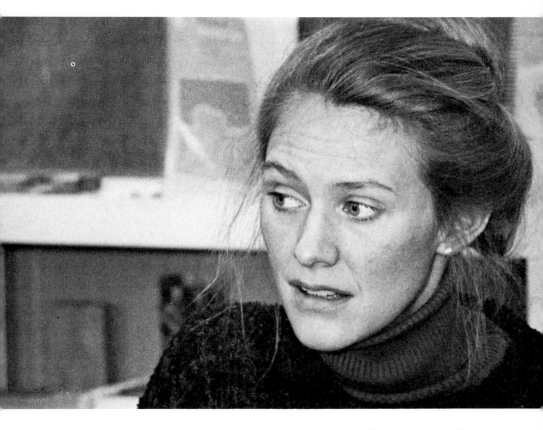

Franci hears that Adrienne cannot receive anything by mouth because of an intestinal problem.

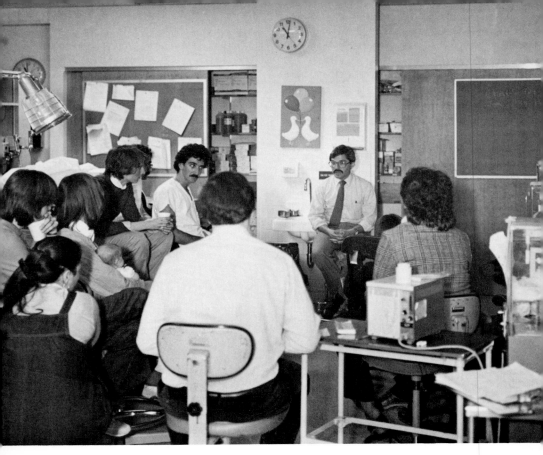

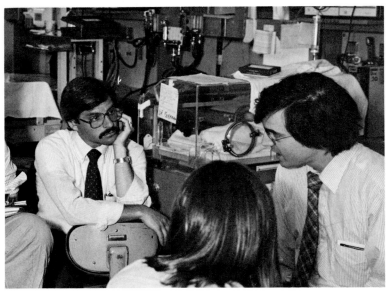

Jaundice

The Webers were puzzled by the bank of bright lights that were over the incubator, and why Adrienne's eyes had to be covered to protect them from the light. Why not turn off the lights if they are so bright? They were told the fluorescent lights helped the baby clear the yellow pigments (jaundice) from the blood. Why did she have jaundice in the first place? Is it serious?

Jaundice refers to the yellow discoloration of the skin resulting from an accumulation of bilirubin (the pigment that produces the yellow color) in the blood, and is most commonly associated with infectious hepatitis or other forms of liver disease in adults. It often comes as a surprise to realize that almost all newborn infants have a little bit of jaundice, which increases in the first days of life, and that this is usually considered "physiological," or so common that it does not carry any serious import. Approximately 5 to 10 percent of all infants born at term will have enough jaundice to attract attention and stimulate a direct measurement of bilirubin in the blood in order to ascertain whether the amount of jaundice deserves some kind of intervention. In other words, a little bit of jaundice is of no significance, but more severe jaundice, as indicated by the rising concentration of bilirubin in the blood, may require treatment. Jaundice can injure the brain of a newborn infant and cause one kind of cerebral palsy.

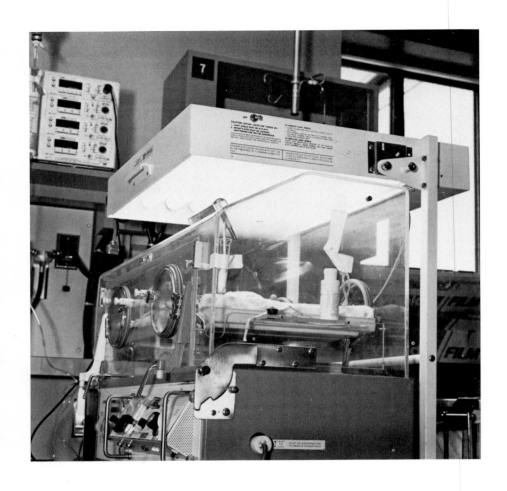

A bank of fluorescent lights provides phototherapy to help make the jaundice less dangerous to Adrienne.

The reasons for the elevation of bilirubin in the blood in the first days after birth are several. First, before birth the infants have to have a high mass of circulating hemoglobin (the pigment in the red blood cells that carries oxygen) because the intrauterine environment has less oxygen than the extrauterine one. Sir Joseph Barcroft, the famed English physiologist, once described intrauterine life as "Mount Everest in utero." The implication is that the infant is at the equivalent of high altitude with respect to availability of oxygen and makes some of the appropriate physiological responses to that environment by increasing the oxygen-carrying capacity in the blood, or, to put it another way, increasing the hemoglobin concentration.

After birth the high hemoglobin concentration is no longer required, since the baby extracts adequate amounts of oxygen from the lungs. The hemoglobin is thus broken down by the body into one of its products, so that one gram of hemoglobin results in the production of 34 milligrams of bilirubin. This load may cause a significant rise in bilirubin concentration in the blood in the second or third day of life.

Another reason for the accumulation of bilirubin in the blood is the inability of the liver of the newborn infant to excrete the bilirubin as well in the first days of life as subsequently.

Not all jaundice is "physiological," and it is important for the physician to think about other possible causes that might require other forms of treatment. For example, if a mother and infant have blood group incompatibility, either from the Rh system or the A, B, O groups, the baby may develop jaundice. In this instance the sequence of events is that some of the baby's red cells enter the maternal circulation during pregnancy and stimulate production of maternal antibodies to those red cells. The antibodies are capable of crossing the placenta in the other direction to enter the fetal circulation and may result in dissolution, or lysis, of the baby's own red cells. Thus, babies with Rh or A, B, O incompatibility may be born anemic, and if the red cell destruction continues there may be a rapid increase in bilirubin in the blood. In fact, the most common cause of jaundice in the first day of life is blood-group incompatibility. In contrast, visible jaundice of the "physiological" type most commonly occurs on the second or third day of life.

When the jaundice is of early onset or when it is more green than orange in color, it suggests the possibility of an obstruction in the liver or bile ducts. This is most commonly related to infection with some degree of hepatitis, which can occur with other kinds of liver disease. The green coloration of the bilirubin reflects its partial metabolism by the liver, with production of other breakdown products. Liver disease in association with jaundice requires investigation for evidence of infection that could have been acquired before birth, even though the mother may never have been aware of having been ill. Rubella (German measles) is a well-known example; during a rubella epidemic a mother may never have felt sick herself, although measurement of antibodies in her blood reveals that she had what is called a "subclinical" infection. The infant, if infected in the first weeks of pregnancy, is at great risk of major congenital malformations. If the mother has the disease toward the end of her pregnancy, the baby risks infection, which can involve the liver and thus be associated with some degree of jaundice. Some of the laboratory studies on blood samples are required to rule out the causes of jaundice that require specific treatment, such as infection.

The treatment of jaundice when it is in the early phases is usually phototherapy. Banks of fluorescent lights are placed over the infant, who is unclothed and therefore capable of absorbing light through the skin. The light converts the bilirubin into its harmless breakdown products by a process called photo-oxidation. The pigments are more readily excreted by the liver and the degree of jaundice is lessened when infants are so treated. Sometimes in the course of phototherapy the babies have a rash reminiscent of small mosquito bites, but this subsides shortly after it is discontinued. Infants under the light also may have loose stools and increased water loss, which can be compensated for by increasing their fluid intake. Sometimes they seem lethargic during phototherapy. When the treatment is no longer necessary, they become more responsive and active.

Exchange transfusions or replacement transfusions may be used whenever there is a need to remove something, such as bilirubin, that is circulating in the baby's blood over a short period of time. The procedure usually involves the insertion of a small catheter into the umbilical vein to provide access to the baby's inferior vena cava (major abdominal vein); blood is withdrawn in quantities of 10 to 20 cc at a time and fresh blood compatible with the baby's own cells is given alternately with the withdrawal. Usually about a pint of blood is exchanged, and thereafter the baby immediately improves because some of the bilirubin has been removed, as well as the red cells that could break down and produce more bilirubin. The baby has been given a good store of red cells that won't be broken down. Sometimes babies require more than one exchange, because the method of alternately withdrawing and injecting blood produces only partial replacement.

If the jaundice is caused by bacterial infection, then of course the babies will require intravenous administration of antibiotics. The reason for preferring an intravenous rather than an oral or intramuscular route is that the gastrointestinal tract of the baby is easily upset, and one can never be assured that antibiotics administered by mouth will not be spit out or vomited or not absorbed by the baby's intestines. The intramuscular route is rarely used because the baby's muscle mass is rather small and one doesn't want to inject potentially irritating substances into such small areas. The intravenous route is far less disturbing to the baby and guarantees the appropriate blood levels of the drug. It is the best way of being assured that the medication is delivered to the site of infection.

In summary: jaundice is very common in the first days of life, particularly in premature infants. Usually it will clear in a week or so without any treatment. Since it can result from a number of causes, and can be severe, pediatricians feel obligated to search for the cause, so that appropriate treatment can be instituted. The use of "lights" or exchange transfusion is undertaken to halt further rise in bilirubin from whatever cause to prevent the possibility of injury to the brain from bilirubin.

This may seem a long-winded discourse for anxious parents. Some, such as the Webers, are curious and want to know more about the problems. Other parents wish the doctors would not burden them with a "lecture." Doctors don't always communicate appropriately!

The news for the Webers was good. Adrienne did not have a significant rise in bilirubin because the lights were effective. They were discontinued on the fifth day of life.

CAT Scan

One of the anxious moments for the Webers took place on the third day, when a CAT scan of Adrienne's head was ordered by the doctor. "We knew that was a test to see if she had bled into her head, and we wondered why it was needed," Mark commented. The CAT (computerized axial tomography) scan is an X-ray study that permits visualization of the spaces, or ventricles, in the brain that contain cerebrospinal fluid.

Very small premature infants have brains that are not fully formed. Blood vessels near the ventricles of the brain are poorly supported by surrounding tissue. Some bleeding occurs in about half of the babies as small as Adrienne and is called intraventricular hemorrhage (IVH). In some babies the fontanelle (the soft spot on the head) bulges because of the bleeding, and the infants may have breathing irregularities or go into shock. In others the CAT scan shows the blood in the ventricles even though the fontanelle does not bulge. If the bleeding continues, or the blood clots, the normal circulation of spinal fluid can be altered and the head may enlarge from the pressure. This problem, hydrocephalus, may require relief of pressure by periodic removal of spinal fluid by spinal taps, or by insertion of a tube that shunts the spinal fluid around the obstruction. Sometimes the blood resorbs and the circulation of spinal fluid becomes normal even without treatment.

In general, a CAT scan is performed when there is a change in the infant's condition, such as slowing or cessation of respiration, because it is the most sensitive indicator of blood in the ventricles. Thereafter, ultrasound is used to follow the course of ventricular size. Since it does not require X-rays, it is considered a safer method for serial studies to evaluate the effect of bleeding.

It is not surprising that the outlook for an infant who has had bleeding into the ventricles relates to how much bleeding there was. It is usually felt that prompt recognition of hemorrhage and prevention of increase in intracranial pressure, along with general supportive care of the infant, will minimize any permanent damage. The association of a previous episode of asphyxia with intra-cranial hemorrhage makes it hard to know whether any late damage is related to the associated asphyxia or the hemorrhage itself. Certainly there is reason for concern when any baby has had intracranial bleeding, but there is no way to predict the consequences to a given infant at the time of the bleeding in the first days of life.

A search for evidence of bleeding into the ventricles is routine on the second or third day of life in all infants as small as Adrienne. She was one of the fortunate ones. Her scan was normal.

3

Intensive Care

First entering a neonatal intensive care unit is like stepping onto a gently revolving carousel. The colored lights of an array of machines blink on and off. There is an endless movement of the staff as they circle the dozen incubators in constant attendance. Beeps and hums and phone rings sound in the background. A parade of metal poles bears a hanging garden of intravenous bottles and tubes.

All this equipment, all these people focus on a single purpose: the nurture of very small human beings who lie virtually motionless in their temperature-controlled chambers, attached to assorted wires and tubes that connect them to the life-supporting machinery.

As Franci and Mark became more comfortable in the neonatal nursery, they became curious about the equipment — the oxygen blender, oxygen monitor, heat shields, and respirators (ventilators).

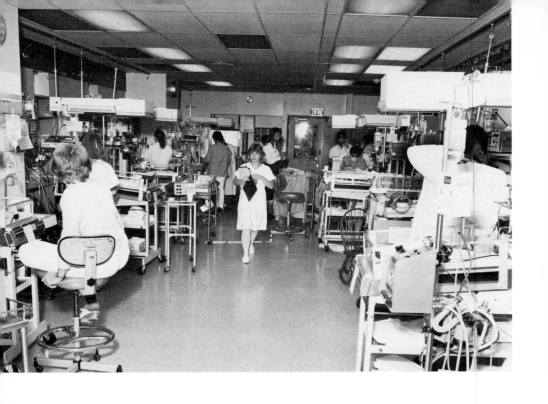

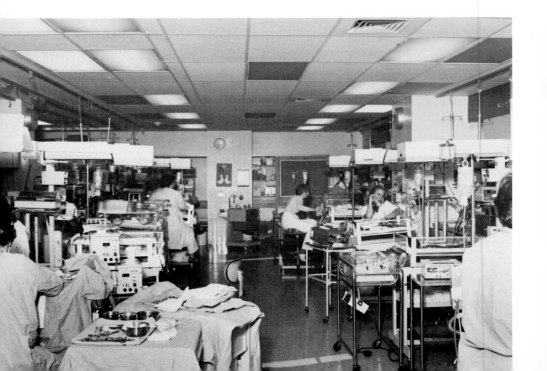

The Webers wondered why Adrienne needed a respirator. Initially she had had to be resuscitated, then she had breathed on her own. Within a few hours of birth, however, it was obvious she did not have the strength to continue regular respirations. As her oxygen needs increased while she failed to eliminate adequate amounts of carbon dioxide, the decision was made to assist her breathing. It was apparent from the pressure required to move air, and her oxygen requirements, that her lungs were more mature than those of most babies her size, presumably because Franci had received the full course of dexamethasone before delivery. The drug had accelerated Adrienne's lung maturation. Thus she had only minimal respiratory distress from hyaline membrane disease.

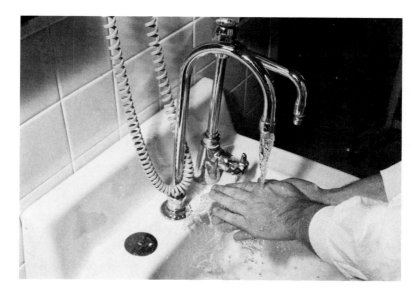

Hand-washing before entering the nursery and before and after touching a baby reduces the likelihood of introducing infection. A gown is worn when an individual plans to touch a baby.

Hyaline Membrane Disease

Hyaline membrane disease has received much attention in recent years, and understanding some ways to prevent it and better ways to treat it has reduced the number of deaths from it. In the 1950s and 1960s about 10,000 premature babies died of hyaline membrane disease and its complications each year in the United States. Now it is estimated that less than half that number die. It is rarely fatal for infants with birth weights over 1500 grams (3 pounds 5 ounces). The smaller the baby, however, the more serious the outlook.

One of the advances has been prenatal diagnosis. Small samples of amniotic fluid can be aspirated through a needle inserted into the uterus by the obstetrician before delivery. This process of sampling the fluid is known as amniocentesis. The fluid can be examined for the presence of a substance called surfactant, derived from the baby's lungs, which has been secreted into the surrounding amniotic fluid. One component of surfactant, called lecithin, is a chemical that the lung requires to function normally after birth. If it is there in appropriate quantities, the lung is mature. If it is deficient, the infant may have hyaline membrane disease. The values for lecithin are expressed as a ratio of lecithin to sphingomyelin, another chemical that does not change significantly during the last part of pregnancy. The lecithin-sphingomyelin ratio (L/S ratio) is usually under 2 in infants at risk of hyaline membrane disease.

When the L/S ratio is low, and it is possible to postpone delivery 48 hours with drugs that quiet contractions, it is sometimes useful to give the mother a drug that will accelerate lung maturity. The drugs are called glucocorticoids, which are hormones or their synthetic analogues, used to mimic the process that would occur

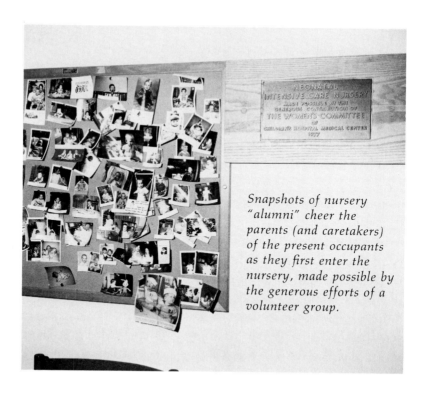

Snapshots of nursery "alumni" cheer the parents (and caretakers) of the present occupants as they first enter the nursery, made possible by the generous efforts of a volunteer group.

naturally if the pregnancy could continue. Dexamethasone, which Franci received, is one such widely used drug. Prenatal glucocorticoids have been shown to reduce the incidence of hyaline membrane disease by two thirds, but they do not always succeed. For reasons yet unexplained, the benefit is somewhat greater for girls than for boys.

Hyaline membrane disease is characterized by unstable lungs, or in other words lungs that tend to go to airlessness on exhalation instead of retaining air, as is normal. The tendency to airlessness, or atelectasis, results from a deficiency of the appropriate phospholipids that normally line the terminal air sacs, called pulmonary surfactant. Surfactant may be deficient at the time of birth from immaturity, or it may be present in reduced amount and used up in the first hours of life.

Coincident with the poor aeration of the lung is a need for increased inspired oxygen. Lack of oxygen further complicates matters by producing constriction of the pulmonary arteries and a tendency for the blood that should go to the lung to bypass it by way of the still open, or patent, fetal blood vessel called the ductus arteriosus (see page 69).

Hyaline membrane disease is treated by using a mechanical ventilator with pressures applied to the airway to oppose the tendency of the lung to become airless. This is called positive end-expiratory pressure (PEEP) or continuous distending airway pressure (CDAP) — sometimes continuous positive airway pressure (CPAP). The pressure can be applied through nasal prongs or through a nasotracheal or orotracheal tube, with or without a respirator. Very small infants, such as Adrienne, also have poorly developed respiratory muscles and usually need assisted ventilation, or IMV (intermittent mechanical ventilation), or require full dependence on a respirator.

In its milder forms, hyaline membrane disease is fully reversible in a few days as the lungs acquire the ability to synthesize the components of the surfactants. When it is more severe, dependence on ventilators may persist for weeks. Sometimes there is a degree of lung scarring, but even this tends to resolve in subsequent months. We do not know for sure when full recovery occurs; we think most infants have adequate lung function by a year of age, but in some severely affected babies testing in subsequent years may reveal residual problems. These children are susceptible to attacks of bronchiolitis in the first year of life. Later, a few may have a tendency to wheeze with exercise. Not enough infants have been evaluated carefully in later childhood to be certain of the long-term outlook.

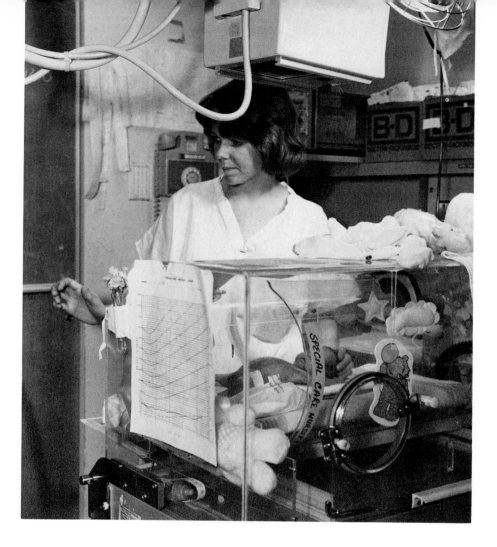

The plastic shell within the incubator (raised temporarily to permit access to Adrienne) is a heat shield. Small infants have a relatively large surface area, which favors heat loss to the environment. They also lack much body fat, which normally provides insulation for the warm body organs. The use of a plastic shell reduces heat losses and permits the baby to be naked so he or she can be carefully observed. The portholes in the incubator permit access to the baby without much heat loss. The chart on the end of the incubator is a growth chart with average weight gains depicted. The uneven line near the bottom shows Adrienne's weight to be near the "expected" value at 51 days of age.

Oxygen Therapy

One of the crucial adjustments the newborn makes at the time of birth consists of breathing air; of bringing in sufficient quantities of oxygen in exchange for carbon dioxide. It is hardly surprising that many infants require added inspired oxygen in the first hours and days of life. Premature infants in particular may require increased oxygen concentrations for weeks or even months. Thus they need to have a device that regulates the amounts of oxygen inspired and other kinds of apparatus to measure the amounts circulating in the blood.

The goal of oxygen therapy is to provide appropriate concentrations in the blood. The risks of too little oxygen, of course, are inadequate supplies to tissues and the accumulation of acids in the body, often called metabolic acidosis. The consequences of excessive oxygen are possible injury to the eyes (retrolental fibroplasia) and the lungs (bronchopulmonary dysplasia).

Added oxygen is given to the baby by increasing it in the air the baby breathes, either from the incubator or from a small plastic hood over the baby's head, which allows better control of the oxygen concentration. If the infant is unable to make adequate respiratory movements, of course, the oxygen is delivered through an endotracheal tube with the help of a respirator.

The adequacy of oxygen in the blood is assessed by serial sampling of small amounts of blood, usually taken from the umbilical artery but sometimes from the radial artery (in the arm) or even the temporal artery (on the side of the scalp). It is possible to make these measurements on just a few drops of blood so that frequent sampling is possible without risk of depriving the infant

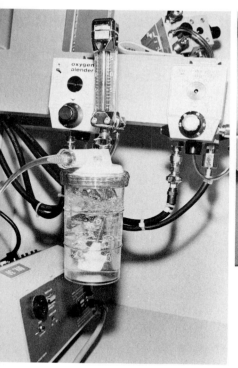
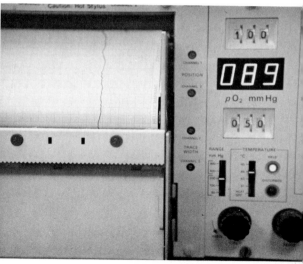

(Left) Oxygen from the wall outlet is blended with room air to the desired concentration and humidified by being bubbled through water before delivery to the infant by way of the plastic tube to the ventilator.

(Right) On the oxygen monitor, the dial reads 89 mm Hg (millimeters of mercury), or partial pressure of oxygen, in the arterial blood as sensed through the skin by a warmed oxygen electrode attached to Adrienne's chest. The graph on the left provides a continuous record of blood oxygen concentration. Very careful adjustment of inspired oxygen is required to keep the baby optimally (but not excessively) oxygenated. Values between 50 and 100 mm Hg are usually appropriate.

of much-needed blood. If many samples are required, not only for measurements of oxygen but for other compounds in the blood, the babies are sometimes given fresh blood transfusions to compensate for the blood loss incurred by careful monitoring of the blood's constituents.

In recent years, it has been possible to have an indirect measure of the oxygen in the blood that reduces the requirement for direct sampling. The device is called a transcutaneous oxygen monitor, which has been shown to give a very accurate assessment of the concentration of oxygen in the arterial blood when the infant's blood circulation is adequate. It is usual to attach the oxygen sensor over the thorax or liver area. This small sensor has a heating element that raises skin temperature to 43–45 degrees centigrade. The heat dilates the small capillary vessels underneath so as to accelerate the blood flow through them, making capillary blood flow the equivalent of arterial blood with respect to its oxygen content. A small polarographic electrode is inserted into the warmer and the oxygen tension across the skin is recorded with the aid of an electronic amplifier, and either a digital or continuous written record. The site of sampling is usually rotated since some slight redness of the skin tends to occur under the electrode. If it is not rotated, a small blister may develop. These small superficial burns resolve in a few days and leave no scarring if the electrode has not been left in the same spot for more than a few hours.

It is important to explain to parents the need for the wires and patches they see attached to their baby. Parents also need the reassurance that the red spots on the skin at the site of the electrode are like a sunburn and will disappear in time.

Umbilical Catheters

Through her first two weeks, Adrienne had a catheter in her umbilical artery. A small, pliable, plastic tube with a blunted tip can be passed into the umbilical artery and on into the aorta to permit the taking of small samples of blood from the baby to measure oxygen and carbon dioxide content.

This procedure would not be done in an infant who was well or in whom use of oxygen was not anticipated. However, many very low birth-weight infants will require oxygen and mechanical ventilation and the insertion of an indwelling catheter is a common practice.

There are some risks associated with an umbilical artery catheter, reported in approximately 1 to 8 percent of babies. The manifestations are usually transient and reversible, although some serious complications have been reported. For example, it is not uncommon for one leg to turn pale transiently from reduced circulation that results from arterial spasm or a small clot located in an artery. Occasionally, small clots can form around the tip of the catheter and these can break loose and restrict the blood supply to the intestinal tract, the kidney, or either leg.

If the catheter is left in place for several days, it is possible to have some redness of the skin around the umbilicus, and occasionally generalized infection can be attributed to the catheter. This hazard increases the longer the indwelling catheter is required.

Sometimes the catheter is placed in the umbilical vein and pushed in through the vessels in the liver to the inferior vena cava. Catheters in this location are needed for exchange transfusion and occasionally for fluid infusion in infants who are in shock and in whom other blood vessels are collapsed and hence hard to use. Many kinds

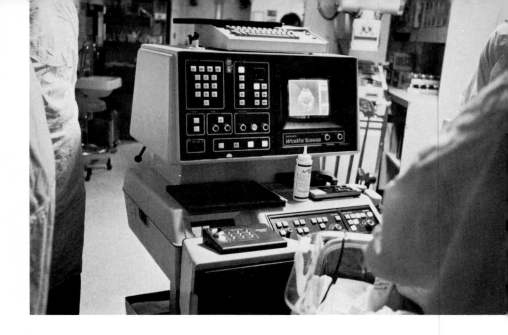

Diagnostic ultrasound allows the cardiologist to see reflections of Adrienne's heart chambers and valves, although they are not easily recognizable to those unfamiliar with this technique. This test is "noninvasive" since the sensor is placed on the skin over the heart. It has replaced more dangerous procedures, such as heart catheterization, in some instances. The test is used when there is a suspicion of patent ductus or other heart problems.

of complications have been associated with catheters in the venous system, including infection and clots. In recent years these complications have been reduced since such a catheter is left in place usually for only a few days. By then one would hope the baby would have stabilized to permit the insertion of a needle in a more peripheral vein.

Occasionally catheters are placed in the radial artery or a needle is placed in a temporal artery. Usually catheters or needles in these locations are used for periodic sampling of blood rather than infusion of nutrients.

Once in a while, when the baby is dependent on intravenous infusion of nutrients, the needle will become displaced and the materials will enter the tissues just under the skin. Ordinarily this is a rare event and people looking after the baby will stop the infusion and replace the catheter more appropriately. Sometimes some of the materials in the intravenous fluids are irritating, however, and injury to the skin, and tissues under it, around the end of the catheter can occur. Usually these injuries can be minimized by careful attention to the catheter, but on occasion the skin will be injured and will require later plastic surgery for an improved cosmetic result.

It is well to remember that no one puts a catheter or a needle in a vein or artery of a baby unless the value of the information to be gained is considered greater than the potential risk. On the other hand, with any invasive procedure a complication can occur.

The Possibility of a Heart Operation

Before birth, the infant receives oxygen and nutrients from the placenta and delivers carbon dioxide and metabolic waste products to it. The placenta, or after-birth, thus serves as a fetal lung, intestinal tract, and kidney. When the umbilical cord is cut, the infant must redirect the circulation to the lung within minutes in order to bring oxygen to the blood and remove carbon dioxide. A series of complex changes take place, but perhaps most dramatic among them is the spontaneous closure of the blood vessel between the pulmonary artery and the aorta that serves as a shunt — the ductus arteriosus. When it closes, blood from the right side of the heart must go to the lung, where gas exchange takes place. If it does not close promptly, blood can bypass the lung and produce cyanosis, a bluish discoloration of skin and mucous membranes.

When infants are born as early as Adrienne, the muscle in the wall of the duct may not be fully developed or responsive to closure by oxygen. After two or three days of life, when the pulmonary blood vessels fully open, the blood may flow from the aorta to the pulmonary artery (the reverse of the direction before birth). If this happens, the lungs may retain fluid and become less compliant, and gas exchange is impaired. These events are reflected in increased oxygen requirements and higher respirator pressures. The heart rate may increase, and the contour of the heart changes, as seen by X-ray examination or ultrasound studies.

In the past infants sometimes died of this complication of premature birth. Now, with careful monitoring of oxygen needs and heart function, the diagnosis of patent ductus can be made. Until a few years ago the only way to close the vessel was through surgery. In 1976 the first cautious reports of the use of a drug, indomethacin, to close the duct were published. Subsequent extensive experience has shown it to be effective most, but not all, of the time. Adrienne, who had symptoms of a patent ductus in the first week of life, was one of the fortunate ones whose improvement was evident one day after she received the drug. Her parents were thus spared the anxiety of waiting through a heart operation on their very small baby. The operation is still needed for a few infants, however, and some of the events that take place are shown in photographs of another infant.

One of the reasons for prompt closure of the ductus is to lessen possible lung damage from the use of high ventilator pressures and high inspired oxygen concentrations. Some infants acquire chronic lung disease in association with these interventions.

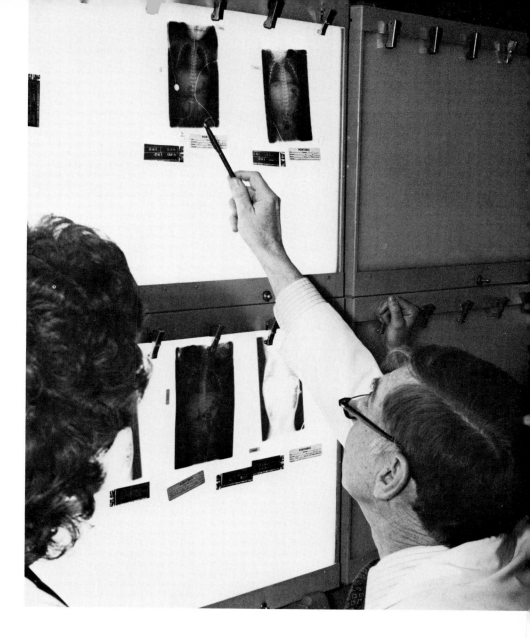

Dr. John Kirkpatrick makes radiology rounds. The chest films are actual size. Small patients have small films.

The lung condition is called bronchopulmonary dysplasia, or, in the jargon of the nursery, BPD. Some infants with BPD require ventilation for more than a month, which is longer than would have been the case in uncomplicated hyaline membrane disease. It is a paradox that interventions that can save life in the first few days, namely the ventilator and the oxygen, also can contribute to injury to the lung that in turn requires their prolonged use, albeit at lower pressures and gradually reduced levels of oxygen. This problem illustrates some of the great difficulties encountered in caring for these infants. It is like walking on a tightrope, or at least treading a narrow path between dangerous alternatives — Scylla and Charybdis.

OPPOSITE
Some babies require an operation to close the ductus arteriosus. A large incision is made in the chest, as shown in this picture of another baby, but it usually leaves only a faint scar in later years.

(Above left)
This is a chest film of an infant at 27 days of age, who had had an operation to close the ductus. The white clip is a device the surgeons placed around the ductus to occlude it. The clip is made of an inert metal, tantalum, and will remain in place for life. It will not have to be replaced. The lungs are still hazy from the effects of this baby's earlier hyaline membrane disease and excess blood from the earlier patent ductus. The infant had a mild form of chronic lung disease called bronchopulmonary dysplasia (BPD). A tube to connect the ventilator with the trachea can be seen in the upper mid-portion of the picture. (PHOTO COURTESY CHILDREN'S HOSPITAL MEDICAL CENTER.)

(Above right)
The tantalum clip is shown beside a pencil to indicate its size.

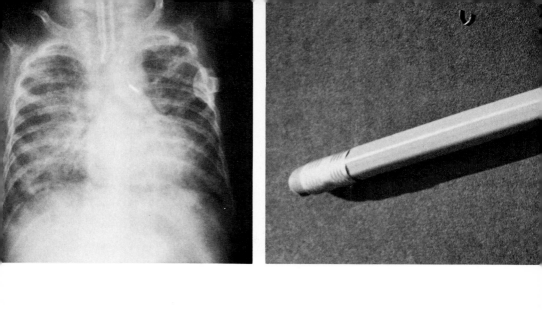

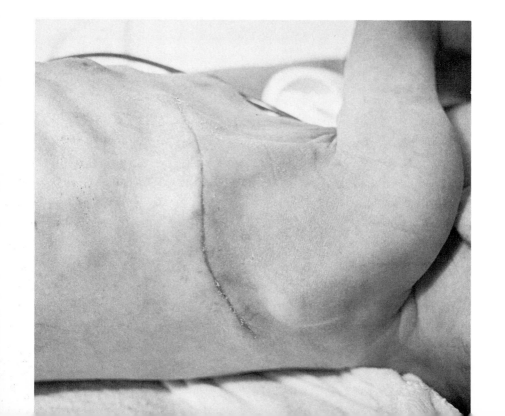

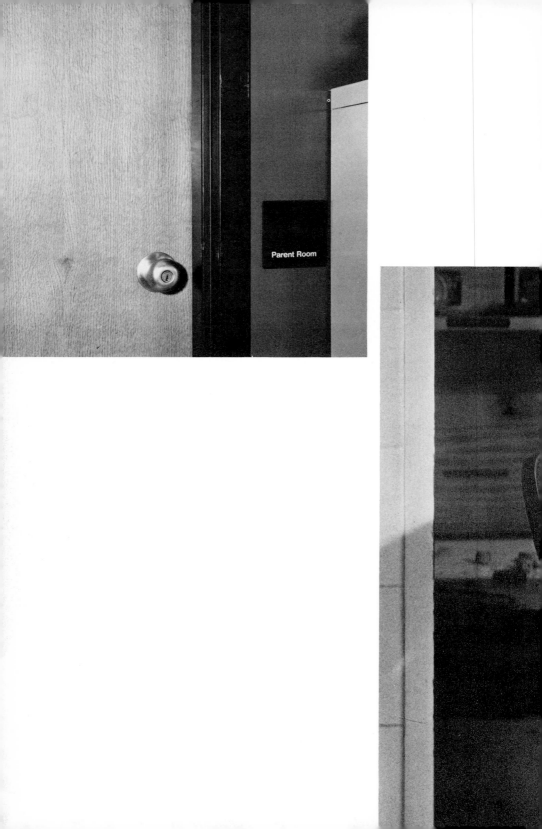

Parent Room

Parents may suffer from "overload" just as the babies can. Franci takes a few minutes to contemplate. What is her responsibility? What is rightfully delegated to the staff? Most important in her mind and in everyone's is what is best for Adrienne.

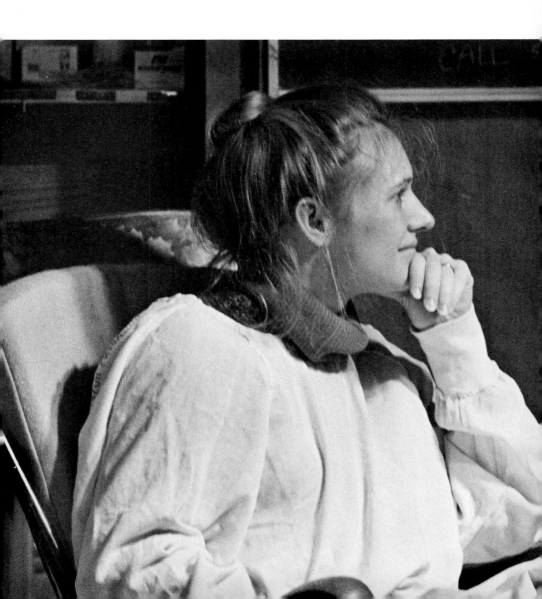

Infant Responses

Those who observe premature infants over many minutes or hours may note the frequency with which they move from quiet sleep to a more active stage of sleep, characterized by an occasional twitch or sucking movements, to wakefulness (even crying), and then back to quiet sleep. They can respond to external stimuli, such as light (by blinking) and sound (by arousal), but soon tire if the stimuli are repeated or excessive. Stroking the infant can have the effect of quieting him, or sometimes it can overstimulate him, as noted by an increase in heart rate and sometimes a change in color of the skin. If the baby experiences stress, he may release adrenaline, which results in mottling of the skin or cooling of the extremities.

Stimulated in part by the studies of Dr. Berry Brazelton and his colleagues, physicians and nurses have learned to be more attentive to the signals the baby sends in response to different and often subtle environmental inputs. One way in which the staff tries to provide a respite from the bright overhead lights is to dim the lights in the whole nursery or in that part where the infants who do not need continuous intensive care can be placed. If that is not feasible, a blanket can be put over the incubator of a given infant at times, to mimic the diurnal-nocturnal cycles of the outside world. Noise levels can be reduced by alerting the staff to the potential for over-stimulation of the babies. Feeding and other interventions are best carried out when the infants are awake, with eyes open, rather than disrupt quiet sleep. The oxygen monitors are very helpful in alerting the caregivers. Painful interventions, overstimulation that can lead to exhaustion, are associated with a fall in the oxygen in the blood. Even a brief rest will allow the infant to return to a quieter state with improved oxygenation.

We do not know how much a premature infant perceives; still, grimaces and withdrawal of limbs may indicate displeasure. Judicious use of pain-killing medication is required for some procedures, and of course anesthesia is used for operations just as in adults. No one pretends it is pleasant to be in intensive care, but every effort is made to minimize the discomfort by giving the infants nipple pacifiers, and by swaddling and stroking them.

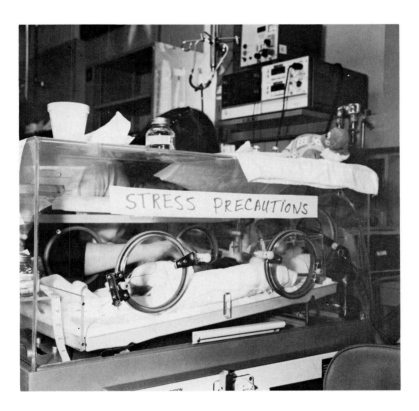

The reminder of "stress precautions" alerts everyone to limit handling of Adrienne to essential needs, and to allow her some rest. The folded diaper over the incubator protects her from the bright lights in the nursery. Intensive care nurseries can be too stimulating at times, and periods of rest are important.

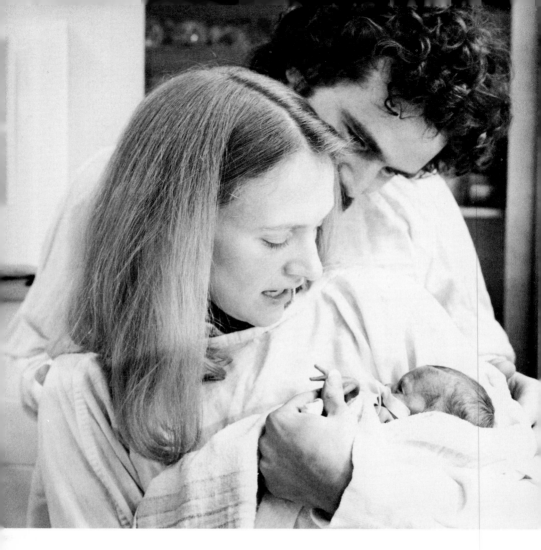

Adrienne at 6 weeks old is able to be out of her incubator and to experience the comfort of her mother's arms and take note of her parents' voices.

By one month of age, Adrienne could be held outside the incubator, although she was still attached to her ventilator. There was no doubt she responded to her parents and her nurses. Infants even on respirators can often be prompted to smile by one month after birth, regardless of how early they were born.

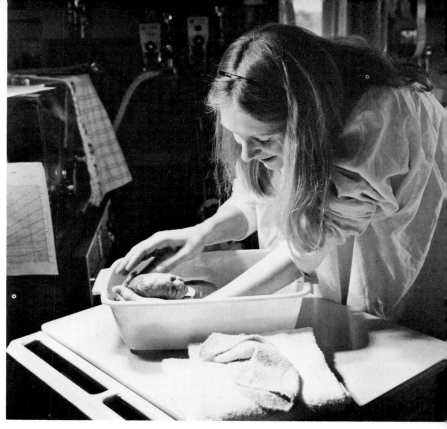

Franci enjoys giving Adrienne a tub bath at 6 weeks.
One of the morning rituals is combing Adrienne's hair with a soft toothbrush. The plastic tube in one nostril ends in the stomach to permit a continuous infusion of small amounts of breast milk since she is still unable to suck sufficiently well to take her feedings by nipple.

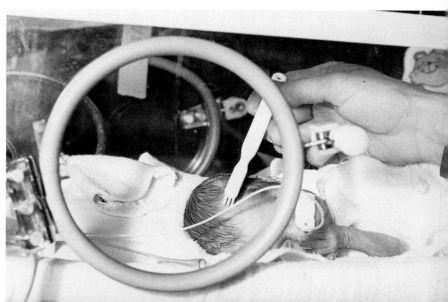

Breathing Irregularities

During the long hours of watching Adrienne through the plastic incubator wall, Franci and Mark often commented on her different patterns of breathing. Sometimes it was perfectly regular, with an occasional deep breath, or gasp. Often it was very irregular when she was awake and moving about. Once in a while she stopped breathing until an alarm went off and someone stimulated her or gave her a few deep breaths with a resuscitation bag.

Most premature infants during their first months of life have a tendency to irregular breathing patterns. When first allowed to breathe spontaneously, Adrienne showed the characteristic bursts of breathing, followed by brief (5-10–second) pauses, then another 10-15–second period of deep breathing, then a pause. Appropriately, this is called *periodic breathing*, and it is accompanied by sucking movements and rapid eye movements.

When the intervals of absent breathing are longer than 10 to 15 seconds, and the heart rate falls, this is designated as an *apneic spell*. An apneic spell is more serious than the much more frequent periodic breathing (without slowing of the heart rate). The heart rates of many infants are monitored by a continuous recording of the electrocardiogram, or ECG. An alarm is triggered by a significant fall in the heart rate (usually to fewer than 100 beats per minute). Gentle stimulation usually restores normal breathing.

One form of gentle stimulation is a water bed, modified for the small infants in a number of ways. A rubber glove partly filled with water and placed under a blanket on which the baby sleeps serves very well. Adrienne rested on such a water bed during much of her time in the incubator when she had a number of apneic spells.

When apneic spells are frequent, more aggressive treatment may be required. Theophylline (a stimulant) or caffeine is sometimes given in small amounts by mouth. The baby needs her "coffee" as much as her caretakers do. This medical stimulation makes respiratory centers in the brain more responsive to the usual breathing stimuli and tends to restore normal patterns of respiration. The diaphragm also contracts with greater force after a small amount of theophylline.

Usually apneic spells become less frequent as the infant matures. Occasionally they persist; if so, a home monitor may be recommended until the infant no longer has further spells. Adrienne did not need one.

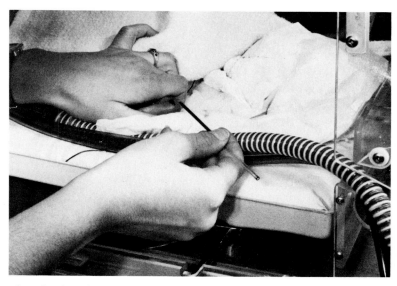

The "heel stick" for a drop of blood is a frequent procedure, considered less difficult than drawing blood from a vein. The blood flows into the capillary tube, or is absorbed onto filter paper for subsequent laboratory tests. All infants have at least one "heel stick" to obtain blood for screening for PKU and other hereditary metabolic diseases. This test is now mandated by law in all states. At other times heel sticks are done to draw blood for measurements of blood counts and blood gases. (The heel is so small it almost looks like the nurse's finger.)

4

Growing Up

The first few weeks of neonatal life are usually the most critical. The complex adjustments from intrauterine to extrauterine life require attention and often assistance. By a few weeks of age attention can be focused on growth and development, and the dependence on ventilators, intravenous nutrition, and monitors can gradually be withdrawn. Babies differ in the timing of their maturation so no single schedule is applicable to all infants.

Adrienne had the most worrisome problems in her first week, with the need for indomethacin to close her patent ductus, and the threat of necrotizing enterocolitis. Her hyaline membrane disease had been mild, but even so she needed some added oxygen for the first two weeks. She required assisted ventilation for 33 days before she could breathe adequately without becoming tired or having apneic spells. Occasional breathing irregularities were noted for two months, so she was kept on theophylline and a water mattress for gentle stimulation.

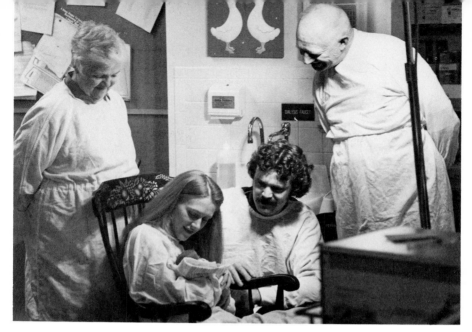

Franci was pleasantly surprised at how immediately her out-of-town parents became attached to Adrienne when they first saw her at 7 weeks. They said about their new granddaughter, "You know, she feels like a good little bundle."

A contented moment.

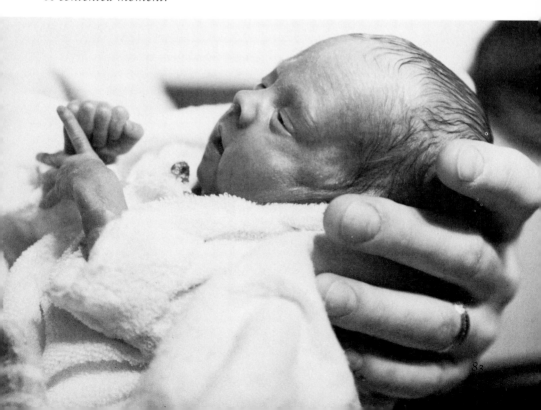

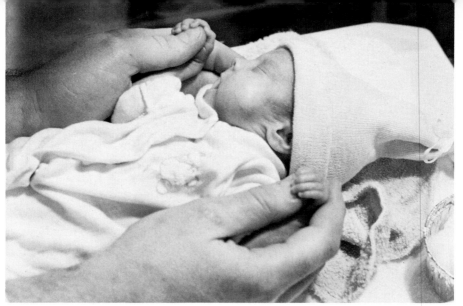

Adrienne's stocking cap helps to prevent heat loss from her skin. Note her fat cheeks, which are common after intravenous feedings. Adrienne grasps her father's thumbs. (Below) Adrienne did not always appreciate her baths. The white disks are left in place for later attachment to the heart rate monitor.

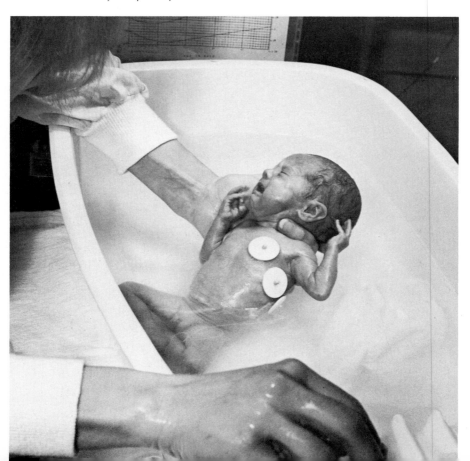

Feeding

Little wonder that on first seeing a small premature infant most parents are concerned about the baby's need to gain weight and grow. Most of a baby's weight gain takes place in the last three months of pregnancy. Birth two to three months early reveals an infant with very little muscle mass and almost no fat. The babies looked starved, but of course they are not. They are at a normal stage of development, but require careful attention to subsequent nutritional needs. Franci noted, "She was so slow to gain weight. I had never expected her to develop without getting bigger." Actually, all infants lose weight after birth, and very small ones require long periods before weight gain is possible. Adrienne's lowest weight was 660 grams (1 pound 7 ounces) when she was 9 days old. She did not regain her birth weight until 19 days after birth. By two months, however, she weighed 940 grams (2 pounds 1 ounce).

During the first days or weeks of life, total intravenous feeding is widely used in the care of small premature infants and others who because of illness may not be able to absorb food from the intestine. Physicians continue to gain experience with intravenous feeding, but still feel the need to measure blood constituents that reflect the amount of body water (hydration) and nutritional status, such as the electrolytes, sodium, potassium, and chloride, as well as some minerals, such as calcium. No two infants are exactly alike, and the composition of the intravenous solutions must be tailored to suit the baby. Parents must wonder why doctors draw blood so often that sometimes they need to replace it with small transfusions of donor blood. The answer is that the knowledge of requirements of babies as small as Adrienne is still incomplete, and careful monitoring is considered essential.

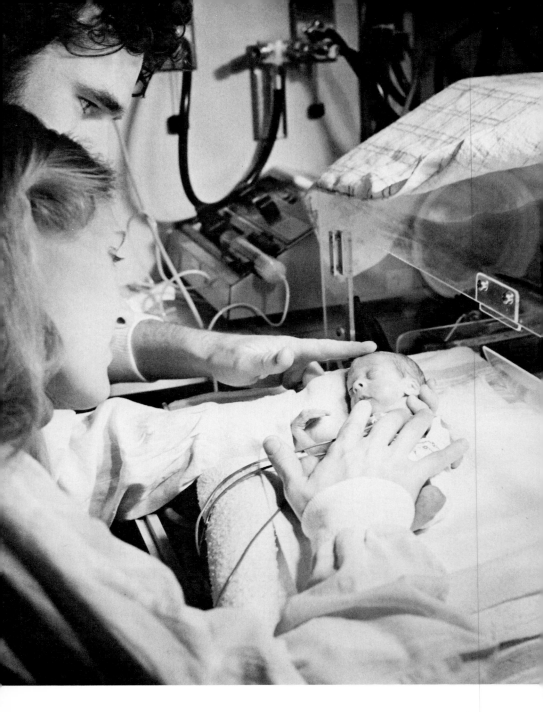

Even though Adrienne is gaining weight each day, at 6 weeks she weighs only 800 grams (1 pound 12 ounces), a net gain of 90 grams (3 ounces) since her birth.

Adrienne was nourished initially through her veins. Later, her mother's breast milk was provided in small amounts through a tube from nose to stomach. By two months she was receiving some milk by mouth from a nipple, and some through the stomach tube. She tired too easily to obtain all she needed by nipple. The nurse had oxygen available in case she turned dusky from breath-holding during feeding.

How much milk an infant can tolerate must be decided on an individual basis. Initially, nutrients are provided intravenously since they are not well absorbed from the intestinal tract. Gradually, the amounts given by tube can be increased, and then later the infant sucks from a nipple. Even when fed by tube (gavage feeding), infants should have the opportunity to suck from a nipple. Digestive enzymes and peristalsis are stimulated by the act of sucking. Pacifiers are recommended in the nursery, but after the age of teething they should be discouraged because they may distort the position of the incoming teeth.

Franci was a faithful provider of her breast milk, but since she could not be with Adrienne every three hours, when the baby needed nourishment, Franci used the mechanical breast pump six times a day. This made it possible for her to produce a day's supply, which was then put in sterile containers and kept frozen in the refrigerator. Milk can be kept frozen for a week or even more without loss of the important constituents that help protect a baby from infection. Usually it is preferable to limit storage to a few days. Heating above body temperature, or pasteurization (at 65 degrees C for 30 minutes), destroys some of the bacteriostatic properties of breast milk.

Franci found that she could provide far more milk than Adrienne required and asked if she could give some to the other babies. She had a blood test to see if she could be a milk donor, but the test revealed evidence of a past encounter with serum hepatitis. She was "positive," in other words, for one of the hepatitis markers in her blood. Thus, to her great dismay and anger, she was told that she could not donate milk, nor could she continue to provide milk for Adrienne. But Adrienne was doing well and had been receiving Franci's milk with supplemental intravenous feedings for now more than two months. Why suddenly should the doctors be so concerned? They tested Adrienne's liver function and her blood, and found everything in order. Franci summoned her courage to insist that she continue to provide milk for Adrienne. As tensions mounted and she realized she was in conflict with the staff, a phone call from the consultant in infectious diseases brought news that there were no documented cases of hepatitis acquired by an infant from breast milk. The crisis was over. Adrienne continued to receive and thrive on her mother's milk. By three months it provided all her nutrition.

In general "wet nursing" or breast banking is discouraged. A mother's milk is ideal for her own baby, but may not be optimal for another infant. A given infant and mother may share antibodies to some infections that can be transmitted by breast milk. Another infant may not be so protected. Under some circumstances, however, the physicians will recommend that an infant with feeding problems receive milk from another nursing mother if the baby's own mother is not nursing.

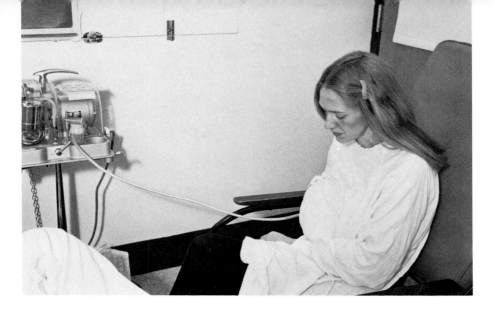

Franci uses an electric breast pump, provided by the hospital, to obtain milk for Adrienne. (Below) Mothers' milk is stored in the nursery refrigerator for later feedings.

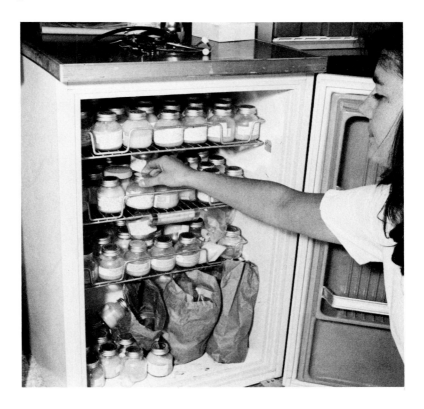

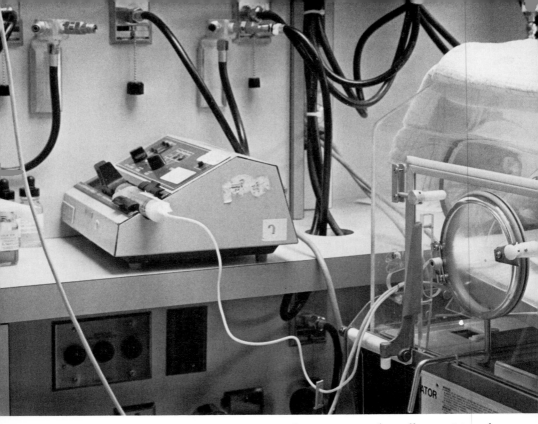

The infusion pump permits continuous administration of small quantities of fluids into a vein. Adrienne, like most very small premature infants, required supplemental nutrients, including sugars, amino acids, and lipids by vein. The lipids make the mixture white so that it looks like milk, but of course it is not. Intravenous alimentation is required whenever the intestinal tract is not able to tolerate normal feedings.

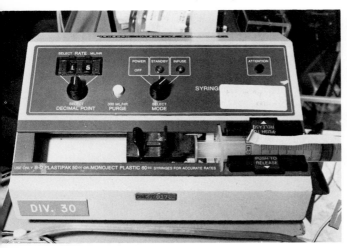

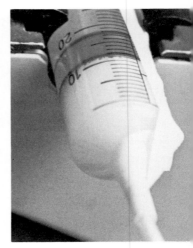

Vitamins

Adrienne was given vitamins to supplement the milk. The Webers wondered why she was given vitamin E (tocopherol) when she was on breast milk. Doesn't mother's milk meet all the needs of the infant in the early months of life?

Adrienne was given vitamin E because infants born prematurely do not derive adequate amounts from breast milk. For example, vitamin E accumulates in the tissues of the infant during pregnancy, so that at five months of gestation the fetus has about 1 mg of tocopherol, and at term about 20 mg. Infants born early are thus deprived of the vitamin E they would have received across the placenta. If it is not provided as a dietary supplement for the first 8 to 10 weeks, infants may have anemia at one to two months of age.

Iron stores are usually adequate until the infant starts to grow rapidly. In general iron is provided by mouth at about two months of age to infants on formula. The adequacy of iron absorption from breast milk varies. Thus it is important to follow the hemoglobin levels in these infants at later visits.

Most premature infants require added calcium and vitamin D to prevent the occurrence of poor bone mineralization and rickets. Here again, the problem is a large demand for calcium when bones are growing rapidly, and inadequate amounts in breast milk or cow's milk to meet that demand. Calcium and vitamin D can be provided as dietary supplements sufficient to prevent rickets. The need is greatest in the first months of life; thereafter amounts in milk are usually adequate.

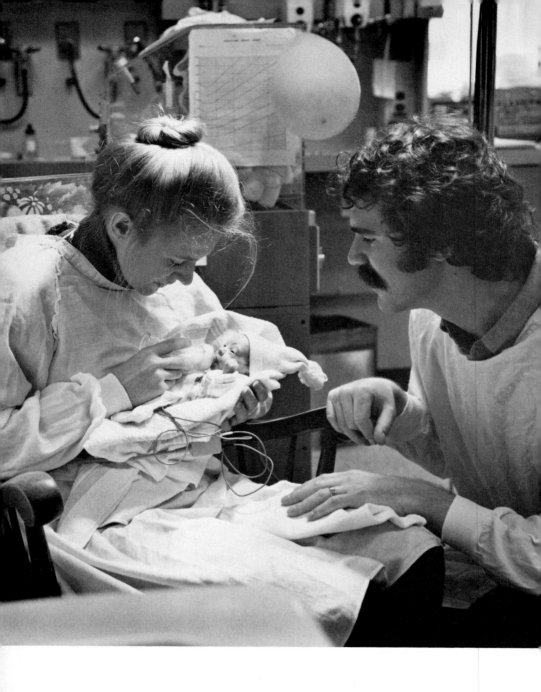

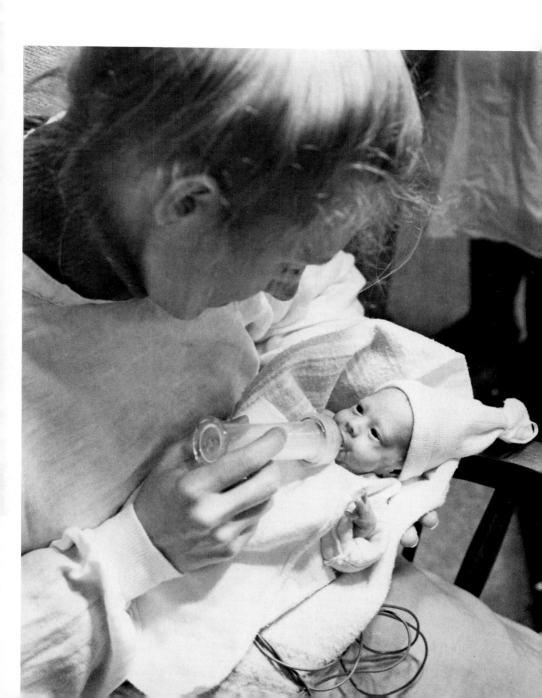

Adrienne, 2 months old, clearly appreciates the breast milk offered by Franci with a bottle.

Vitamin C (ascorbic acid) likewise is required by infants in about the same daily doses as adults need. Before birth, levels of vitamin C in the blood of infants exceed that of the mother. Premature infants require vitamin C to utilize protein required for growth. Although classic vitamin C deficiency (scurvy) is rarely seen in infants, moderate deficiencies lead to an inability to metabolize the amino acid tyrosine. This problem is very common in the presence of excess amino acid (protein) intake or vitamin C deficiency. Infants on prepared formulas will require added vitamin C. Breast milk usually contains adequate amounts.

Folate, the salt of one of the vitamin B groups, folacin, is usually present in higher concentrations in the fetus than in the mother. Premature infants have low serum folate levels unless they receive it in their formulas. Lack of folate interferes with red blood cell production in the bone marrow, which is most evident in the second and third months. The white blood cells are also affected, the most common finding being a change in the shape of their nuclei, called hypersegmentation.

Breast milk is allowed to flow by gravity through a thin plastic tube inserted through the mouth into the stomach. This is called gavage feeding and is used when the infant is too weak to suck.

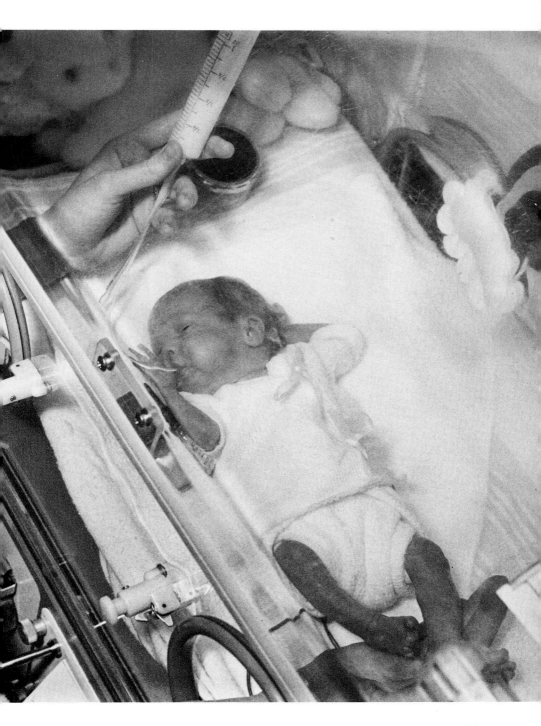

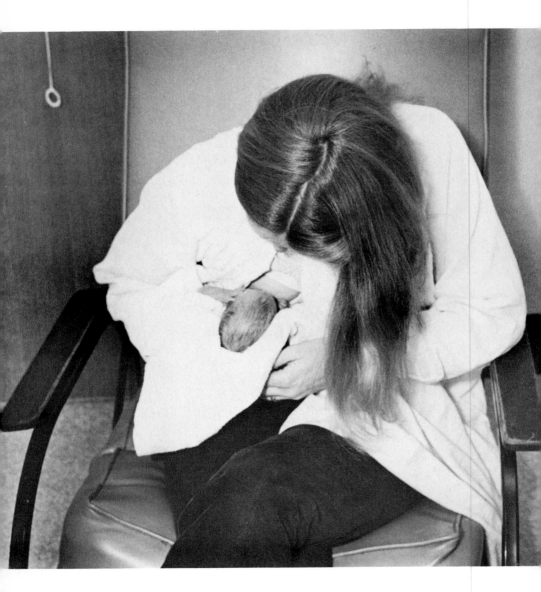

Adrienne could suck a little milk from the breast by 10 weeks of age, but required gavage feedings to complete her daily requirements.

<small>OPPOSITE</small>
The possibility that Adrienne may have acquired hepatitis makes necessary this sign on the incubator, on Easter Day.

Medical Records

Sometimes the medical record weighs more than the baby!

Since no single individual can be with an infant 24 hours a day, communication between shifts of doctors and nurses requires a written record of medications, vital signs (temperature, pulse, respirations), oxygen intake, fluid intake, calories, stools, frequency of urination, specific gravity of urine, and comments about activity. Diagnostic procedures are also noted, as well as the infant's tolerance to handling.

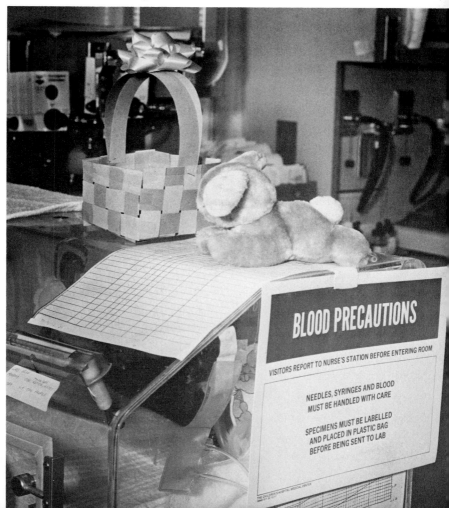

BLOOD PRECAUTIONS

VISITORS REPORT TO NURSE'S STATION BEFORE ENTERING ROOM

NEEDLES, SYRINGES AND BLOOD
MUST BE HANDLED WITH CARE

SPECIMENS MUST BE LABELLED
AND PLACED IN PLASTIC BAG
BEFORE BEING SENT TO LAB

Adrienne's medications were Neo-Calglucon to provide added calcium, vitamin E, folate, potassium, phosphate, Lasix (a diuretic, or drug to help increase urine production). In addition, her feedings were fortified with polycose (a mixture of easily absorbed sugars) and MCT oil (medium-chain triglycerides) to provide added calories without fluid overload. Her total intake was 150 cc per kilogram of body weight per day, and her caloric intake was 134 calories per kilogram per day, or about the same amount per kilogram as an infant born at term would get. On this formula her weight gain was 20 grams per kilogram per day, which was appropriate for her postnatal age.

Adrienne, 11 weeks after birth. The bandage on the heel marks the site of an earlier blood test.

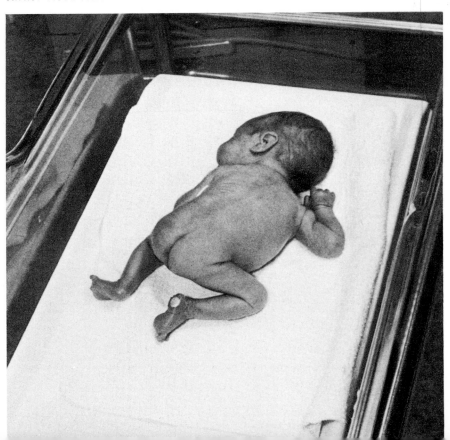

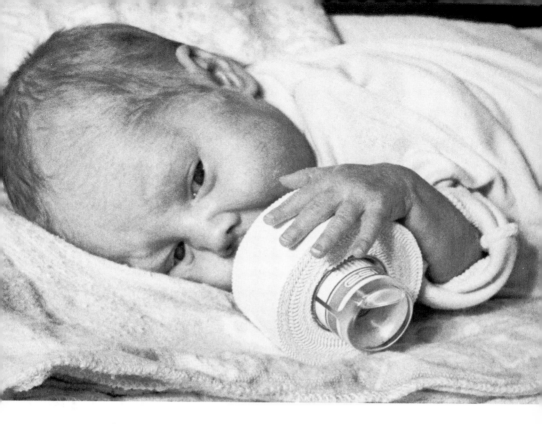

Adrienne, age 11 weeks, is encouraged to suck on a pacifier, which stimulates salivary and gastric secretions and provides comfort. The bandage around the bottle makes it easier for her to hold.

The daily notations of formula changes, medications, recording of results of blood tests, and observations of Adrienne's responses by doctors and nurses generated the voluminous notes that comprised her "medical record."

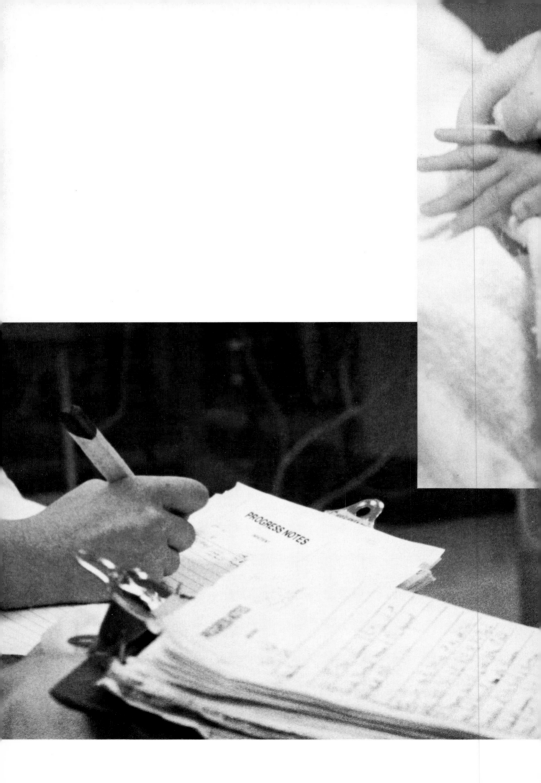

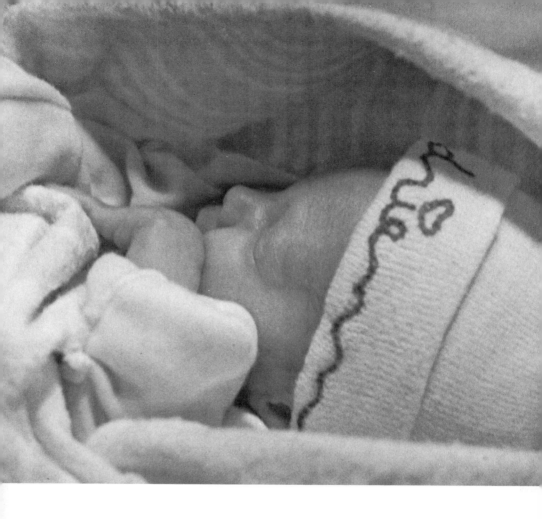

Doctors and nurses keep careful written records of events important in the care of Adrienne. Vital signs — temperature, heart
rate, respiration rate, and blood pressure — are noted, as well as
ventilator settings, concentration of oxygen required, and administration of intravenous fluids and drugs hour by hour. These notations become part of the progress notes that eventually will make
up Adrienne's permanent medical record.

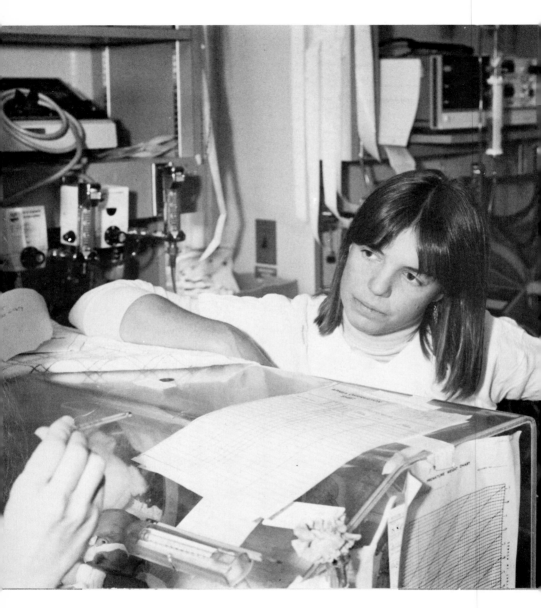

Dr. Pamela Fischer confers with a nurse about Adrienne's temperature.

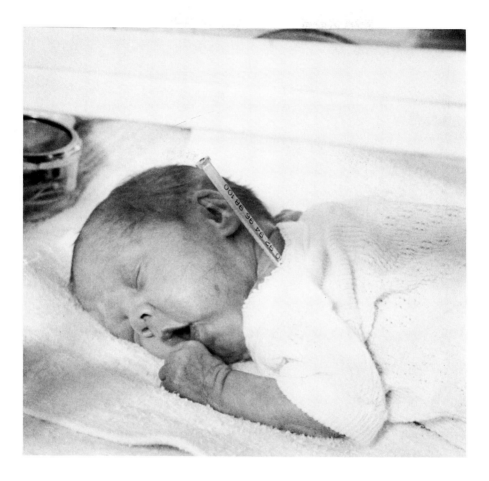

Adrienne's temperature is measured by a thermometer placed under her arm.

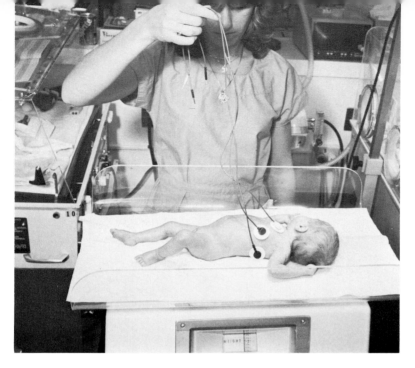

Daily weights are measured without the addition of the monitoring equipment. Adrienne at 109 days old weighs 1280 grams (2 lbs 13 oz). The weight of the sheets and the ECG leads is subtracted to give Adrienne's real weight.

Adrienne is moved temporarily to a crib during a change of incubator, and measuring her length is part of nursery "routines."

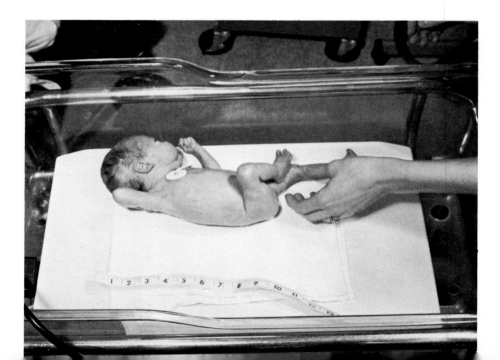

5

At the Beth Israel Hospital

Once Adrienne could breathe without assistance of a ventilator, and grow without dependence on intravenous nutrition, the decision was made that she no longer needed "intensive care." Even though she wasn't ready to go home, her needs could be met in a less frenetic environment, where there were fewer nurses and less sick infants.

So the move back to the Beth Israel Hospital was another milestone, recognition of Adrienne's ability to do well in a new setting. Franci was pleased because she had returned to work as an obstetric nurse-practitioner part-time, and was frequently in the Beth Israel Hospital with her own patients. Her many friends in that hospital became a "cheering section" for little Adrienne. Franci admitted to some apprehension about the move before it happened, because she had come to know and trust the staff at Children's. Change often raises anxieties.

The move required putting Adrienne into a "transport incubator" complete with portable power pack and oxygen. Accompanied by a doctor and nurse, Adrienne rode in the ambulance for one block, to her birthplace, while Mark and Franci walked to Beth Israel.

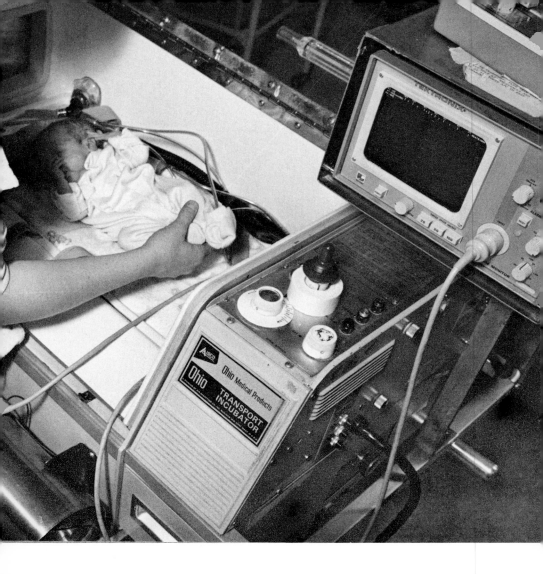

The transport incubator is almost a nursery on wheels, complete with oxygen, suction, heat, and devices for monitoring the heart rate. Most important, however, is the presence of her primary nurse, who was familiar with her every move.

OPPOSITE

(Top) The transport incubator comes equipped with a portable gas tank (the white oblong tank attached to the carriage). Note also the small oscilloscope on top of the incubator to permit monitoring of the electrocardiogram during transport (shown also in the preceding picture). (Bottom) Adrienne is lifted into the ambulance.

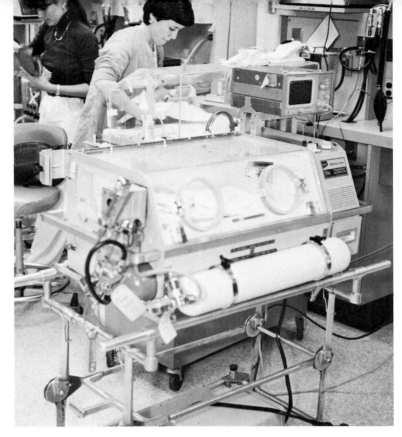

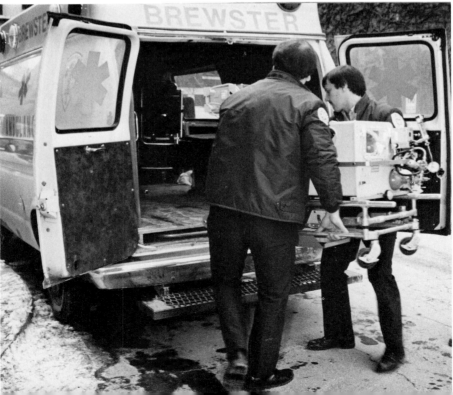

An important aspect of regionalization of intensive care is the ability to put the infants who need the most intensive care in one setting (sometimes called a level III nursery). When the needs of the baby can be met with fewer staff, and no crises are expected, nurturing care can be provided in a less intense environment, called a level II nursery. Adrienne continued to need close watching, but was now free of her dependence on high technology equipment; thus the move to Beth Israel's level II nursery at 82 days of age.

When she was 13 weeks old, Adrienne was moved from an incubator to a crib. The previous week the incubator temperature was lowered by keeping the portholes open, and Adrienne was clothed in a shirt, diaper, cap, and booties. When it was evident she could maintain her own body temperature at normal levels in the surrounding, or ambient, room temperature, she was moved to the crib. Now she weighed nearly 4 pounds.

The tolerance of small infants to room temperature varies with their size, postnatal age, and body fat reserves. Rarely is it possible to move them from the incubator before they weigh 1400 grams (3 pounds 2 ounces) and are on full oral feedings. More commonly they are placed in cribs when they weigh more than 1600 grams. One of the most impressive observations is that subcutaneous fat, measured as a skin-fold thickness, increases in infants at room temperature compared with that of babies kept at the warmer incubator temperatures. In other respects, such as weight gain, no significant differences have been noted.

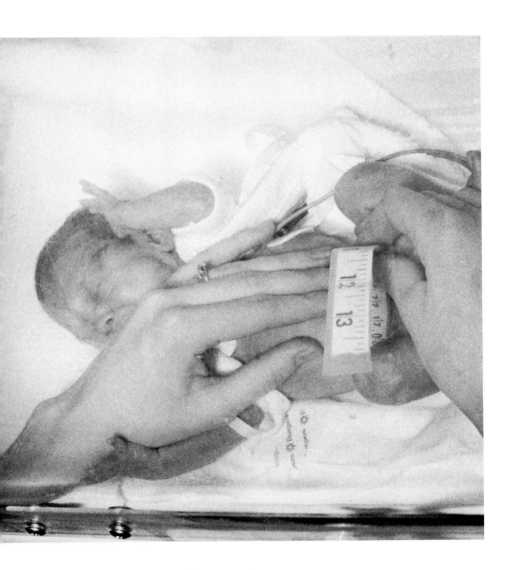

Abdominal girth requires frequent measurement.

Retrolental Fibroplasia

One week after the move, on May 1, 1982, when Adrienne was three months old (but still before the estimated date of delivery), the ophthalmologist saw the mild changes of retrolental fibroplasia (RLF) in both eyes. There was at that time no evidence of resolution.

Retrolental fibroplasia, first described in 1942, is an abnormal mass of scar tissue that forms in the eyes of premature infants. It may be very mild and of little significance, or it may be of such an extent that it displaces the retina of the eye and causes blindness. Indeed, in the early 1950s it was the leading cause of blindness in this country.

Infants most at risk of retrolental fibroplasia are those of low birth weight and short gestational age. The more immature the developing retina of the eye, the greater the susceptibility to this condition. Although oxygen is surely one factor in causing the disease, some infants, particularly those of very low birth weight, have had RLF in the absence of a high oxygen environment. Very careful monitoring of blood oxygen to avoid too much or too little is one of the most important ingredients of neonatal intensive care, and has surely been associated with a reduction in the incidence of RLF in recent years. Blindness rarely occurs in infants over 3 pounds birth weight, but infants as small as Adrienne may still have visual loss even with the most meticulous attention to oxygen concentrations.

The changes can usually be detected at six weeks to several months of age. The abnormal proliferating blood vessels are best seen with indirect ophthalmoscopy. (Since this has been used only in recent years, it may account for a greater recognition of retrolental fibroplasia.)

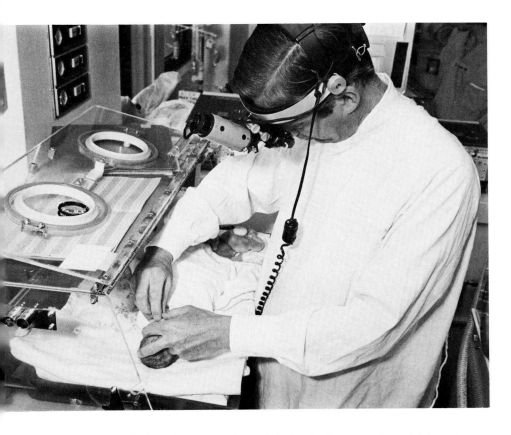

Dr. Robert Petersen, the ophthalmologist, examines Adrienne's eyes with an indirect ophthalmoscope to check on the retrolental fibroplasia. One hand steadies the head, the other lifts the eyelid.

Franci and Mark were told there was a chance that Adrienne might be blind. No one could tell for sure. All they could do was hope she had the reversible kind of lesion. As the next month went by, it was clear once again that she was one of the fortunate ones. On discharge home her eye examination was normal.

Franci and Mark continued their daily visits. Franci went back to work part-time but admitted Adrienne was on her mind very often. "The first thing I did when I woke up was to phone the nurses and find out how her night had been." Mark, too, found he was bringing daily reports to his fellow office workers. "They feel this is their baby, too. The mother of one of the secretaries wants a day-by-day accounting of how she is doing. I brought in some pictures and Emily insisted she borrow a couple to show her mother." Franci added, "We have probably gotten more phone calls since Adrienne was born than we had in the last two years before that."

Visiting was a pleasure, but had a problem. Mark said the nurses occasionally made him feel guilty when he left. "When are you coming back?" one asked, and Mark found himself making excuses for leaving Adrienne. Franci added that sometimes she got the impression that if she did not stay with Adrienne she was perceived as an uncaring mother. Perhaps nursery personnel sometimes overdo the open visiting policy. Parents have their rights, too.

The Webers expressed the feelings common among most parents of premature infants. No one wants a pregnancy to end early. Everyone has some anxiety about the future of an infant who requires intensive care for the first months of life. It often helps to discuss these perfectly normal concerns with the staff and other parents. Complete assurance of a normal outcome is never possible. The focus has to be on the many small events of each day. Parents become part of the "cheering section" for their infant, and work with the staff to meet the needs of their infant in the ways in which they are most comfortable.

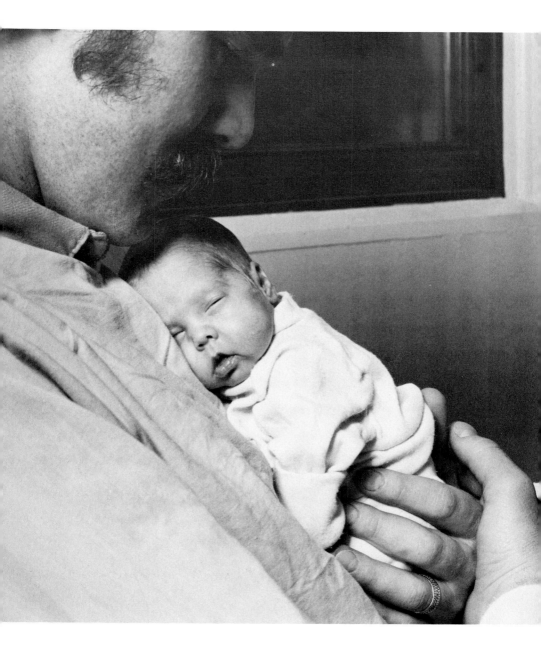

Mark enjoys his daily vists with Adrienne, and she finds relaxation at these times, too.

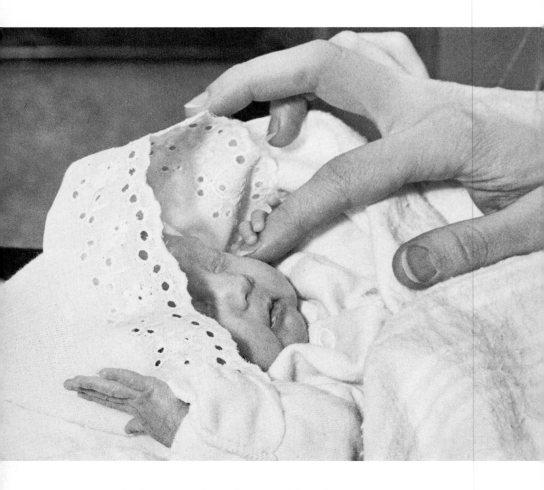

Franci made the bonnet for Adrienne, although it functions more as a "light shade" right now. Mother and daughter share a moment of love.

About 10 percent of infants born weighing less than 1500 grams (3 pounds 5 ounces) will have some hearing loss. If the infant does not respond normally to two tests, some special attention to communicating with the baby will be helpful, such as speaking clearly and louder than normal with the infant watching the speaker. Consultation with experts in infant speech and hearing is appropriate. Hearing aids can be used even in the first year of life if needed. Adrienne's reponses to the bell and to other hearing tests are normal.

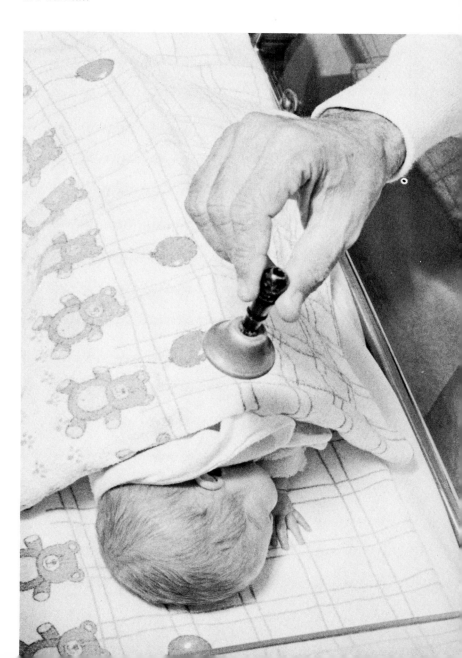

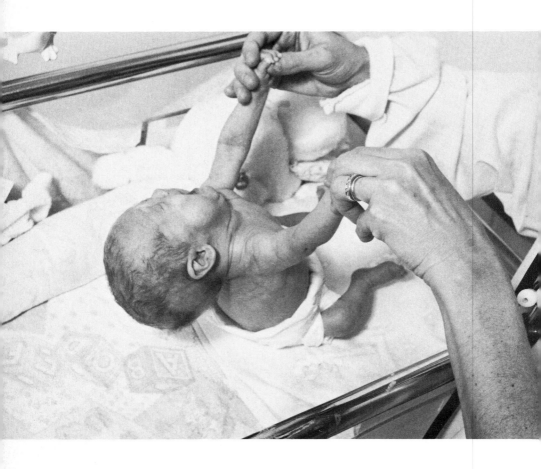

At 16 weeks of age Adrienne cannot quite manage to lift her head.
It is well to remember, however, that this is just about the time
she was due to be born. Her postconceptual age is 40 weeks. Frequently during the days of growing up, the staff tests the infant's
responses to light and sound, as well as muscle coordination. It is
useful to note the developmental milestones.

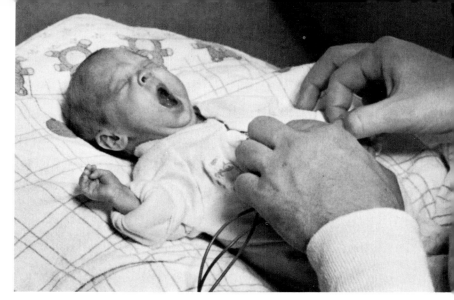

Even a premature infant can find life boring.

The pacifier diverts Adrienne from the blood test.

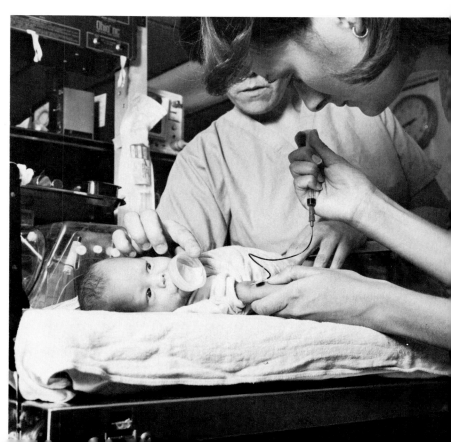

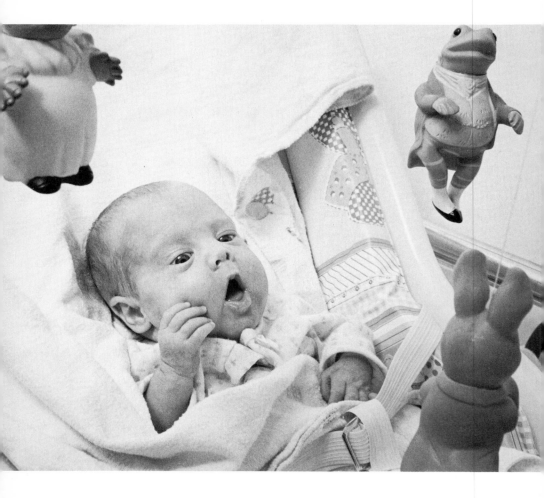

Adrienne is surprised when her mobile moves.

6

Going Home

After a few weeks of adjustment to life in a crib, in contrast to an incubator, the question arises as to the most appropriate time for discharge home. When weight gain has been steady and no problems have required medical intervention, the infant has demonstrated that all probably will go well at home. In general, discharge does not occur before the date the baby would have been at term.

The timing has to be negotiated with the parents. Since Franci had been nursing Adrienne, she was delighted at the thought of having her nearby for every feeding instead of pumping her milk for others to administer. However, she discovered she was to have little sleep at first since Adrienne preferred to be fed every three hours.

Adrienne had a developmental evaluation that showed her abilities to meet expectations, given her very premature birth. A hearing test (auditory evoked potentials) was also normal. Blood studies showed she was mildly anemic, which is not unusual in premature infants.

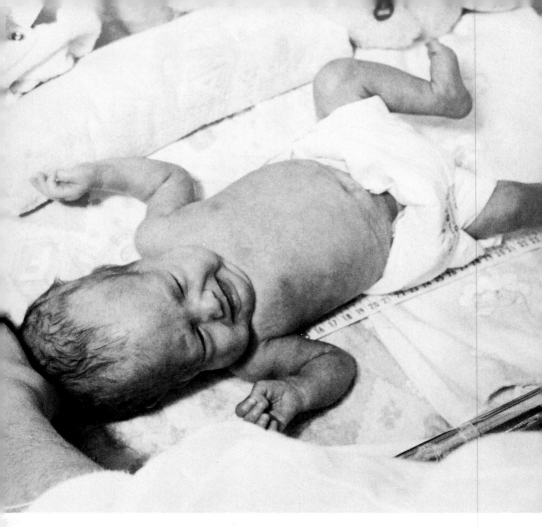

At her discharge physical examination Adrienne is 39 centimeters (nearly 16 inches) long, almost 7 centimeters longer than when she was born.

Plans were made for a visit to her pediatrician one week later to check the blood count. Every examination provided reassurance that Adrienne was ready for discharge, even though she weighed only 1960 grams (4 pounds 5 ounces). Though she was 16 weeks old, she was one week post-term, or one week beyond her mother's due date when she went home, on May 19, 1982.

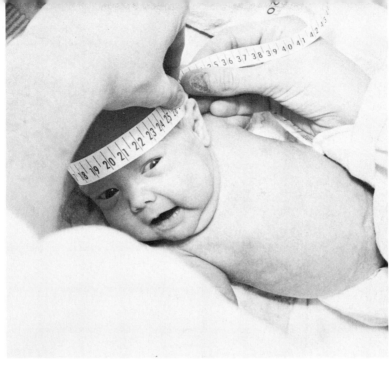

Serial measurements of head circumference are a good indicator of brain growth. Disposable tape measures ensure against contamination and possible cross-infection. At 16 weeks, Adrienne's head is growing at an appropriate rate, which is reassuring in light of the ever-present possibility that an earlier episode of bleeding in the ventricles of the brain might have been overlooked.

The doctor checks her heart at the discharge examination.

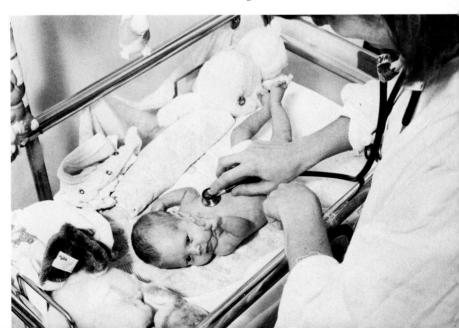

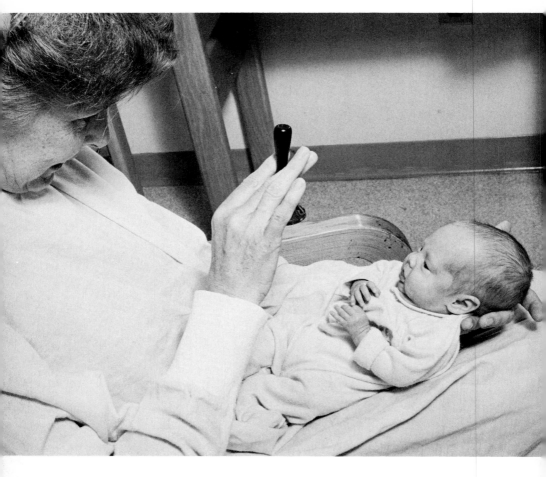

By now Adrienne is interested in the sound of the bell.

This is the day of celebration. The nurses have marked the event by writing "Going Home" on her stocking cap.

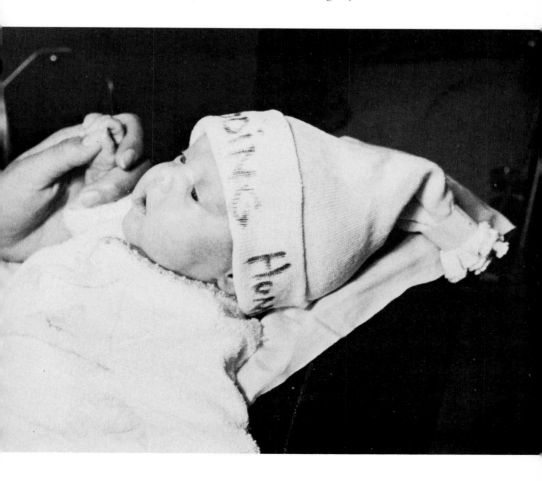

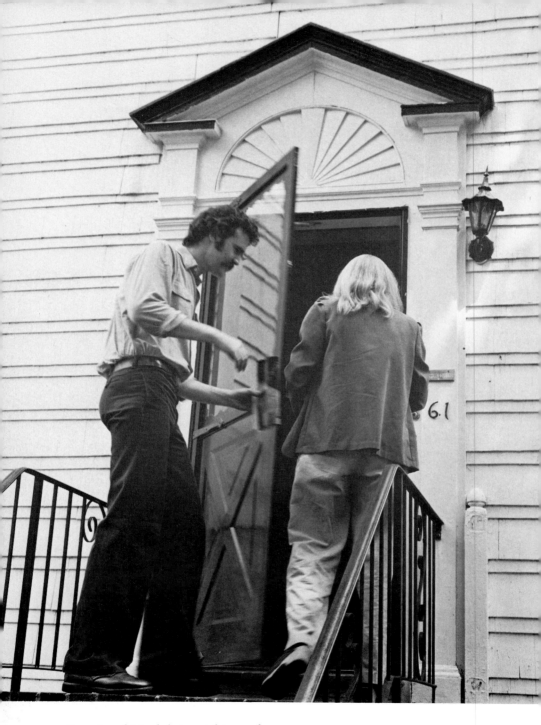

Franci and Mark bring Adrienne home.

Getting acquainted with a new baby at home always brings some excitement, and often some anxiety. These natural reactions are exaggerated when parents realize they now must assume the responsibilities that formerly had been shared with the hospital staff. Each day's experience brought a little more confidence, and Adrienne seemed undisturbed by the new setting.

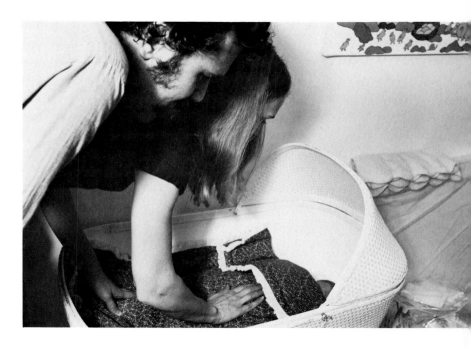

Adrienne is ready for a nap in her very own cradle.

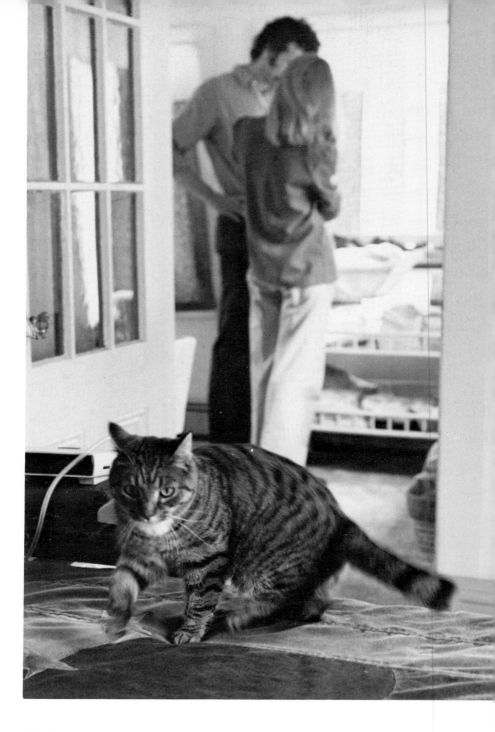

The family cat was not forewarned of the turn of events.

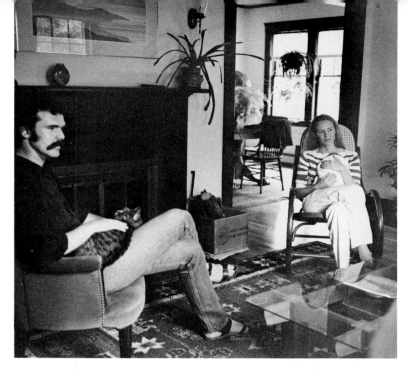

During a visit three days later, Adrienne sleeps, while the cat is consoled by Mark.

Sleepy baby, proud father.

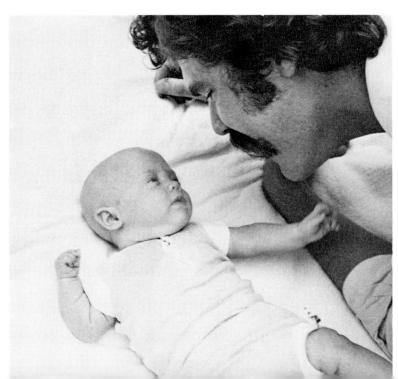

Having stopped working part-time, Franci quickly settled into her new routine. She was reasonably sure Adrienne was doing well, but confided that she was somewhat tense before the one-week checkup with her pediatrician. Would she have gained enough weight? Would her responses be appropriate? These perfectly normal questions cannot always be answered with certainty because most pediatricians have never had patients of such low birth weight who have received modern intensive care. A guarded answer to many questions may be justified, but at the same time it may induce unnecessary anxieties. In general, each day marks some progress, which should be noted on its own terms. Long-term prognostication is usually unnecessary.

One common question is how to measure age. Is it from the birth or from the day of expected birth? Of course birthdays will mark the day of actual birth. Adrienne's doctors will apply an age-correction to her growth and development and speak of conceptual age when they assess her later performance. Thus, from the developmental perspective Adrienne was about two weeks old at the time of her discharge.

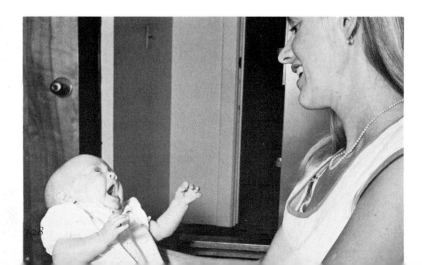

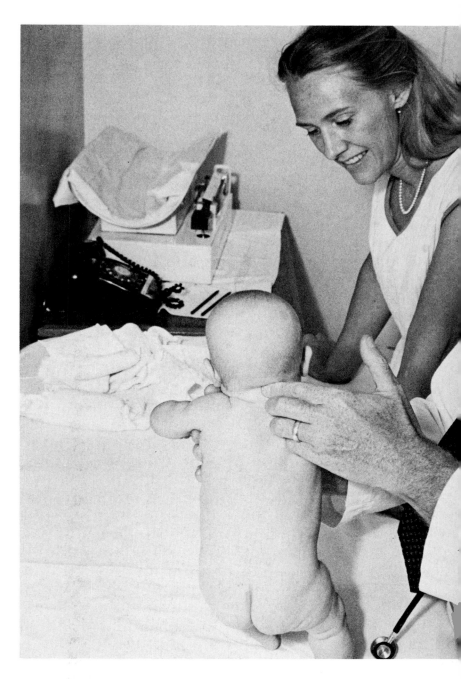

Franci looks forward to a visit every month with her pediatrician, and Adrienne, at 27 weeks, shares in the delight.

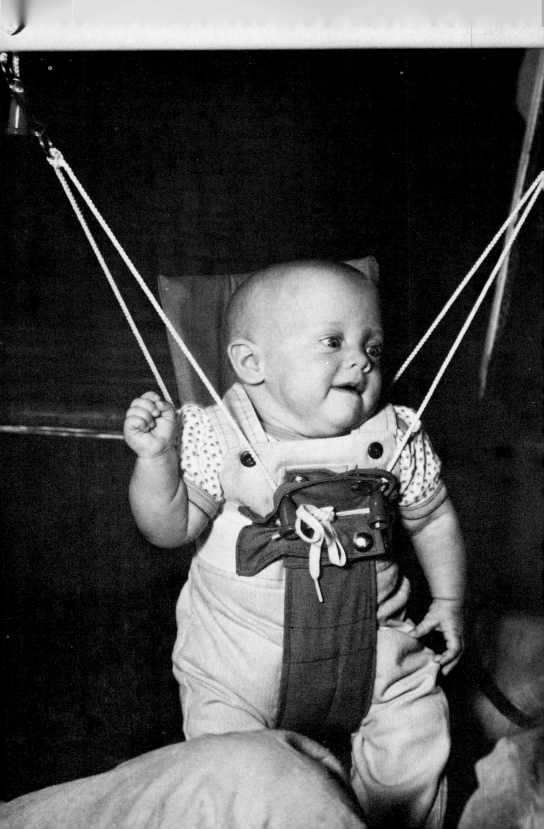

How long must one consider two different ages for the same infant? The answer is, when they converge or, in other words, when "catch-up" is complete. The time of convergence differs as a function of the degree of prematurity. Neurological maturation may be precocious in some respects when premature infants are compared to newly born term infants of like weight. They act as if they have had some practice in relating to others, which of course is true. Weight, on the other hand, may lag for six or more months, so that a very small infant at three months post–due date will probably be smaller than an infant three months after term birth.

In general, a baby doubles birth weight by four to five months, and triples it by a year. Adrienne almost tripled her birth weight of 710 grams by three and one-half months after birth. She was in the process of "catch-up growth" but would require a few more months to become indistinguishable from infants born at term.

When Adrienne was six months old (but only two months past term), she could lift her head when pulled to a sitting position. A week later she burst into a broad smile and thereafter seemed to enjoy her newly found achievements. Parents often can note weak smiles and obvious contentment from a much earlier age. Indeed, the nursery nurses were certain Adrienne smiled during her first month of life. A wide grin in response to a stimulus comes much later. Franci noted that "real smile" in mid–July 1982.

Adrienne, nearly 6 months old, enjoys a summer afternoon.

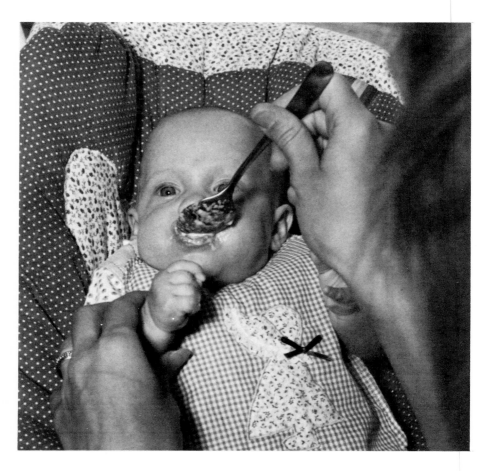

This is her first solid food.

During the summer months Franci took Adrienne with her on trips to the store. She thought of Adrienne as six months old, but because she weighed only nine pounds, strangers would assume she was much younger. One day a stranger told Franci she should not take the baby out without a cap. Another saw Adrienne yawn, and suggested Franci take her home and give her a nap. Franci commented she thought she would be turned in as "awful mother of the year!" Fortunately, Franci's own understanding of the special past history of her daughter made it possible for her to laugh at the gratuitous nature of the comments rather than become upset at her perceived inadequacies. These kinds of events are not unusual and certainly should not prevent parents of premature infants from taking their babies to other homes and even stores. By six months of age Adrienne had acquired most of the attributes that are appropriate for her post-conceptual age of two months. She deserved to be treated like any other two-month-old infant even though she was smaller than most. Franci and Mark had the right idea.

All's well that ends well.

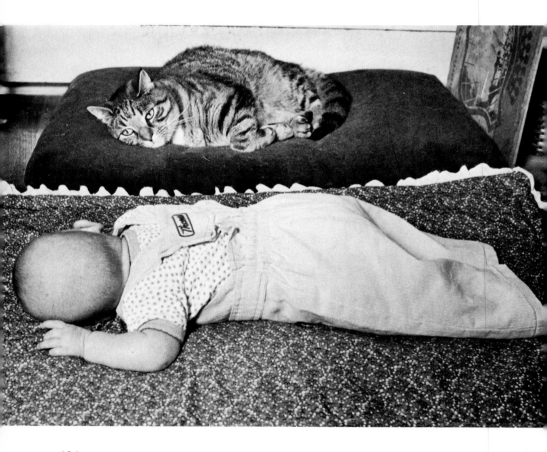

Epilogue

The Webers shared some personal reflections when Adrienne was seven months old, after nearly four months at home.

One of their insights was about the anger they felt about what had happened, and the realization that they directed some of that anger toward each other. "It strained our relationship. We were rarely home together. For the three and a half months of hospitalization, we both wanted to be with Adrienne. We decided to visit separately to avoid competition." When Adrienne was home, they felt for the first time they were, at last, a family. It was a tremendous relief finally to take over and have control.

Franci expressed her tensions during the days of hospitalization as a sense of being in limbo. She wasn't pregnant anymore, but she did not have a baby at home. She was very much alone. The hours with Adrienne in the hospital helped. So did conversations with other parents. Nonetheless, she felt a sense of inadequacy since the "norm" was a big fat baby and she had a very small, fragile one.

These feelings are widely shared by parents of premature infants. Sensitivity on the part of all concerned to the frustration, anger, helplessness, and emotional tensions of parents is a sometimes overlooked part of neonatal intensive care. Although the daily conversation among parents, nurses, and physicians in the intensive care nursery tends to focus on the small details that relate to a given infant, the overriding and often unspoken question concerns the long-term outlook for the child-to-be.

The question is of course very difficult to answer with any certainty. In an effort to be helpful, the staff may volunteer information sometimes unduly pessimistic when it is about a potentially ominous finding, or sometimes unduly optimistic when they wish to be encouraging and supportive rather than realistic. Avoidance of the question may be viewed as poor physician-parent communication. Answers based on the latest medical literature may pertain to a group of infants whose condition and environment differ sufficiently from that of the infant in question to make comparisons invalid. Often the only honest answer must be "we cannot know for sure," or, to quote the words of my own Quaker physician, we must "learn to proceed as the way openeth."

Predictions generally can at least take into account present experiences with survival — meaning discharge home from the nursery — and follow-up through childhood of low birth-weight infants. The table on page 137 shows the percentages of survival at two Boston hospitals for 1977 and the first six months of 1981. The overall impression is that 90 percent of infants weighing over 1500 grams at birth are indistinguishable from infants born after a normal-term pregnancy by two years of age.

Comparison of the Percentage of Surviving Low Birth-Weight Infants (discharged home), 1977 and 1981

Birth weight (gm)	Brigham and Women's Hospital and Beth Israel Hospital	
	1977	1981
500–600	0	14*
601–700	4	14
701–800	23	52
801–900	44	64
901–1000	42	77
1001–1500	87	92
over 1500	99+	99+
Total number of infants under 1500 gm	153	251

---

*Numbers are small. One baby of seven lived.

(The outlook is least good for those least mature at birth, and improves with advancing gestational age at the time of birth.) Among the factors that contribute to late morbidity are a history of asphyxia at birth, major congenital malformations, serious infection before or after birth, prolonged requirements for increased oxygen and mechanical ventilation, and significant intrauterine growth retardation. Individual infants may be normal even in the presence of one or more of these risk factors.

In general, infants who are born early but of appropriate weight for their gestational age show some "catch-up" growth after the first month of life. By the age of one year, they weigh 1 to 2 pounds less than infants born at term and are about one inch shorter, but are still within the normal range for weight and height (see growth charts, pages 150–151). They are noted as being in the tenth percentile; that is, 10 percent of infants born at term will weigh less, and 90 percent will weigh more. Infants who are undersized for their gestational age, or "light for dates," grow at about the same rate as infants of the same size but of appropriate gestational age. They are less likely to "catch up" and tend to remain relatively small throughout childhood. Their ultimate stature depends on a number of factors, the most important of which is the reason for their intrauterine growth retardation. Infants with chromosomal abnormalities or those who had severe infections before birth may be destined to be relatively small throughout life.

Continued attention to the special needs of these infants, and pursuit of the causes and means of prevention of premature birth are the best assurance that the notable progress of recent decades will continue in the years to come.

In a society that is rightfully concerned about escalating costs of medical care, surely readers must wonder about the cost of three and one-half months of hospitalization for Adrienne. The total bill was just over $100,000. The family Blue Cross–Blue Shield policy paid all except part of the ambulance fee for transport. The Webers' out-of-pocket expense was $200.

Must it be that expensive? The largest part of the cost was for the professional personnel whose training and experience made possible the intensive care Adrienne received. The specialized equipment and laboratory tests added significantly to the cost, as did the "overhead" of a special care nursery. Think for a moment of the behind-the-scenes workers who maintained the equipment, prepared the medications, provided the clean environment, and administered the major medical center in which this and many other human dramas occur. We know that in time greater efficiencies can be achieved, and it is one of our ongoing responsibilities to evaluate all interventions from the perspective of efficiency as well as effectiveness.

Meanwhile, we make available the same standard of care for all infants regardless of parents' ability to pay. More than 90 percent of parents have some form of health insurance, including Medicaid. For those who have no insurance, the bills are adjusted according to the family's resources, and payments may extend over years.

Excellent care at the beginning of life is expected to have a seventy-year payoff. The cost of survival with handicaps can far exceed the cost of neonatal intensive care. The human cost of lifelong disability is beyond calculation. We think the value of the investment in Adrienne amortized over her lifetime far exceeds $100,000.

Glossary

For those who hear the medical terms and the verbal shorthand of the intensive care nurseries and seek an explanation.

AMINO ACIDS   Constituents of proteins that can be given intravenously.

AMNIOTIC FLUID   The liquid that surrounds the baby before birth.

ANOMALY   Malformation of an organ.

AORTA   Major blood vessel from the heart.

APNEA   Absence of breathing.

APNEIC SPELLS   Short, often recurrent episodes of cessation of breathing with slowing of the heart rate, usually ending with a deep breath. Babies sometimes need mechanical stimulation (such as a water bed) to keep breathing.

ARTERY   Blood vessel that carries oxygenated blood.

ASPHYXIA   The consequence of lack of oxygen, suffocation.

ATELECTASIS   Airlessness in portions of the lung.

BICARBONATE   One of the constituents of the blood that affects its acidity.

BILI-LITES   Lights, usually fluorescent, placed in a rack above the incubator to help clear the bilirubin by photo-oxidation. Bright daylight does the same thing.

BILIRUBIN   The pigment in the blood that makes the skin yellow. It rises whenever blood is broken down by the body, as occurs in infants in the first days of life. It also rises in some types of liver disease.

BLEED   Usually refers to intraventricular hemorrhage.

BPD   Bronchopulmonary dysplasia. Refers to the late stages of hyaline membrane disease. It is a form of lung injury associated with use of ventilators and oxygen. It may last for weeks or months.

BRADYCARDIA   Slowing of the heart rate.

CAT SCAN   Computerized axial tomography (sometimes called CT scan). This is a procedure using X-ray pictures taken across several planes that are then assembled by computer to distinguish varying densities in the pictured areas. It is the best way to locate blood or other masses in the head.

CATHETER   A hollow tube. Catheters come in different sizes to insert in blood vessels or the bladder, or any site that requires drainage.

CO_2 Carbon dioxide. This product of metabolism is removed through the lung.

CONGENITAL   Present at birth.

CPAP   Continuous positive airway pressure, used to help keep air in the immature lung.

CRIT   *See* Hematocrit.

DES   Diethylstilbestrol, a synthetic analogue of estrogen.

DEXTROSE   A form of glucose (sugar).

DOPPLER   An auditory signal produced by blood in vessels, used to measure blood pressure.

DUCT   Ductus arteriosus. This blood vessel between the aorta and pulmonary artery is open before birth and should close after birth. Sometimes in premature infants it does not close and may require ligation or operation.

ECHO   The use of ultrasound to reflect from tissues in the body (it is based on the same principle as sonar). In the nursery echo, or ultrasound, studies are commonly used to diagnose heart anomalies. Other uses are to detect bleeding in the head or other parts of the body, and abnormal masses in the chest or abdomen.

EDEMA   Swelling (usually from fluid retention).

EEG   Electroencephalogram. It is a measure of the electrical activity of the brain.

EKG OR ECG Electrocardiogram. It is a measure of the electrical activity of the heart.

ELECTROLYTES Constituents of the blood that carry an electrical charge, such as sodium, potassium, and chloride.

ENDOTRACHEAL Inside the windpipe (trachea).

EXTUBATE To remove a tube from a body orifice.

FIO_2 Fraction of inspired oxygen. The FIO_2 of room air is .21, or 21 percent oxygen. An FIO_2 or 1.0 means 100 percent oxygen.

FONTANELLE The soft spot in the center of a baby's scalp. At birth the bones of the head are not fully formed and fused; the fontanelle is the membrane-covered junction between the frontal and parietal bones. Later, the bones will fuse and the fontanelle will disappear. A smaller fontanelle can be felt farther back at the junction of the occipital and parietal bones.

GANGRENE Death of tissue from occlusion of blood flow to it.

GASES Oxygen and carbon dioxide in the arterial blood.

GAVAGE Feeding through a small tube placed through the nose or mouth and ending in the stomach or upper intestine (may be continuous or intermittent). When the route is nose-to-stomach, it is called N-G. When it is nose-to-small intestine (jejunum), it is N-J. When it is mouth-to-stomach, it is O-G or orogastric.

GLUCOSE A simple sugar that can be given intravenously. The amount of glucose in the blood is followed closely, particularly in infants of diabetic mothers or in those who are small for gestational age.

HEMATOCRIT The percent of red cells in the blood. An increased concentration is polycythemia. A decreased concentration is anemia.

HEMOGLOBIN The amount of oxygen-carrying pigment in the blood. A low hemoglobin could be from too few red blood cells, or too low a concentration of hemoglobin in each red cell.

HYALINE MEMBRANE DISEASE (HMD) Also called respiratory distress syndrome (RDS). Immature lungs may be unable to remain aerated when the baby breathes out. The increased respiratory efforts cause some liquid to enter the air spaces. Under the microscope it looks like a membrane, hence the name. It usually clears in a few days. Severely affected infants require ventilators to help keep air in the lungs.

HYDROCEPHALUS Abnormal accumulation of fluid in the head. Excessive pressure from bleeding or abnormalities in the circulation of spinal fluid can lead to a full and tense fontanelle and eventually too rapid head growth.

HYPERALIMENTATION   Provision of nutrients by vein. *Hyper-* usually means in excess of needs. When used as a prefix for alimentation, it implies addition of sufficient quantities to meet needs.

INCUBATOR   The covered plastic device in which infants are placed to help maintain temperature, humidity, and appropriate oxygen concentration.

INFUSION PUMP   A device to push liquids slowly and continuously. It is used in small infants to provide the appropriate amounts of water, salts, and nutrients.

INTRALIPID   A trade name for a mixture of fats derived from soybeans that can be given intravenously.

INTRAVENOUS (i.v.)   Into a vein.

INTRAVENOUS ALIMENTATION   Nutrients given by vein. Very small, weak, or sick infants may not absorb milk from the intestinal tract. Their daily requirements can be met by suitable nutrients given by vein.

INTRAVENTRICULAR HEMORRHAGE (IVH)   Blood in the ventricular system in the center of the brain. Immature infants are particularly susceptible to some bleeding at this site. It often clears spontaneously, but may require treatment.

INTUBATE   To put a tube into the trachea to permit mechanical ventilation.

ISOLETTE   Trade name for incubator.

JAUNDICE   The yellow color seen in the skin when bilirubin is elevated.

LANUGO   The hair over the brow, shoulders, and back present at birth but shed in the subsequent weeks.

LASIX   A drug (diuretic) used to promote excretion of water by the kidneys.

LAVAGE   Rinse.

LP   Lumbar puncture. A needle is inserted into a space between lumbar spinous vertebrae to permit withdrawal of some spinal fluid.

LYTES   Jargon for electrolytes (see above).

MCT OIL   Medium-chain triglycerides, a nutritional supplement.

MECONIUM   The dark green-black viscous material in the bowel of the infant before birth. It is usually passed in the first 24 hours.

MONITORS   Electronic devices to display or record information, such as heart rate, respiratory rate, or oxygen concentration.

NEC   Necrotizing enterocolitis. Immature infants, particularly if they have been asphyxiated or in shock, may have impaired blood supply to portions of the bowel. Small perforations can occur, with air dissecting in the bowel wall or even entering the peritoneal cavity.

NECROSIS   Death of tissue.

NPO   *Nil per os*; Latin phrase meaning "nothing by mouth."

PATENT DUCTUS   The duct that remains open when it would normally be closed; also called PDA.

PAVULON   A muscle relaxant given to some babies who resist mechanical ventilation.

PEEP   Positive end-expiratory pressure (to help keep the lungs aerated).

PERIODIC BREATHING   Five-to-ten-second pauses followed by bursts of breaths. Almost all low birth-weight infants (and some full-term babies) have some respiratory irregularities.

PERSISTENT FETAL CIRCULATION (PFC)   A phrase referring to the constriction of the pulmonary blood vessels often found in infants who have aspirated meconium. Such infants usually require increased concentrations of oxygen to help relax the pulmonary arteries.

pH   Denotes the acidity or alkalinity of the blood. A pH of 7.40 is normal for arterial blood.

PHOTOTHERAPY   Use of light to reduce the level of bilirubin in the blood by photo-oxidation.

PIE   Pulmonary interstitial emphysema (air dissected in the tissue planes of the lung).

PNEUMOTHORAX   Lung rupture with air outside the lung.

P.O.   *Per os*; Latin phrase meaning "by mouth."

PO_2 OR PaO_2 Partial pressure of oxygen in arterial blood. This is a measure of the oxygen that can be delivered to tissues, and should be between 50 and 100 millimeters of mercury.

POLYCOSE   A mixture of easily absorbed sugars.

PULMONARY EDEMA   Excess water in the lung. This can occur for a number of reasons. A major reason is persistent ductus arteriosus, or other forms of heart failure.

RADIAL LINE   A catheter in the radial artery (usually at the wrist).

RESPIRATOR   A device that pushes air into the lung and allows the passive recoil of lungs and chest to push air out after it has exchanged oxygen for carbon dioxide in the lung. Respirators may be called by their trade names, such as Baby Bird, Bourne, Air Shields, etc. They are sometimes referred to as ventilators.

RESPIRATORY DISTRESS SYNDROME (RDS) *See* Hyaline membrane disease.

RETICS Reticulocytes. These are immature red cells and are present in increased number after blood loss or blood destruction.

RETROLENTAL FIBROPLASIA (RLF) Injury to the retina of the eye. The condition occurs in some immature infants (more common the more immature the infant). It is usually detected after some weeks in the nursery. Excessive oxygen is the most common cause, but it can occur in very small infants without a history of receiving oxygen. Mild forms are reversible; severe forms lead to blindness.

SALINE Salt. "Physiological saline" is a solution of 0.9 percent NaCl.

SEPSIS Infection.

STORK BITES This unusual label refers to flat red spots (capillary hemangiomas) that are common over the central forehead above the nose and the nape of the neck. They become less prominent as the skin thickens with age.

SURFACTANT The surface active material that lines the airspaces of the lung to prevent their closure.

TACHYCARDIA Rapid heart rate.

TACHYPNEA Rapid breathing.

THEOPHYLLINE A stimulant drug of the methylxanthine class.

TRANSCUTANEOUS OXYGEN MONITOR A device to measure oxygen in capillary blood under the skin without piercing the skin.

THRUSH The common name for a fungal infection of the mouth. White plaques may appear on the mucous surfaces of the tongue, gums, and throat. The Latin name is *Candida albicans*.

UA LINE Umbilical artery catheter to permit sampling of baby's blood and to measure blood pressure.

UMBILICUS The navel. The placenta is attached to the baby by the umbilical cord, which enters the baby's abdomen at the umbilicus.

VEIN A blood vessel that carries venous blood to the heart.

VENTILATOR *See* Respirator.

VENTRICLES The chambers of the heart or head.

VERNIX The white, greasy material that coats the skin at birth.

VITAL SIGNS   Temperature, pulse, respiratory rate, blood pressure.

WET LUNG   Refers to liquid in the lung that has not resorbed as fast as expected after birth. This condition may also be called transient tachypnea of the newborn, or TTN.

WHITE COUNT   The number of white blood cells (leucocytes) in the blood. This value helps ascertain the presence of infection. Different kinds of white cells are sometimes described separately as polys (polymorphonuclear), monos (monocytes), and lymphs (lymphocytes).

Appendix

Annual Statistics
Conversion Tables
Growth Charts

Annual Statistics
United States

	Total births (in millions)	Total deaths	Live births at less than 2500 gm	Percentage of low birth-weight infants
1968	3,502	56,456	286,500	8.2
1973	3,140	40,664	236,300	7.25
1978	3,333	31,618	236,300	7.1
1981	3,646	26,828	247,900	6.8*

*Provisional.

Note the significant reduction in total deaths in a decade of advances in care of infants. The percentage of low birth-weight infants has shown a modest but encouraging decline.

Conversion of Inches to Centimeters

Inches	cm.	Inches	cm.	Inches	cm.
10	25.40	15	38.10	20	50.80
10½	26.67	15½	39.37	20½	52.07
11	27.94	16	40.64	21	53.34
11½	29.21	16½	41.91	21½	54.61
12	30.48	17	43.18	22	55.88
12½	31.75	17½	44.45	22½	57.15
13	33.02	18	45.72	23	58.42
13½	34.29	18½	46.99	23½	56.69
14	35.56	19	48.26	24	60.96
14½	36.83	19½	49.53		

CONVERSION OF
POUNDS AND OUNCES TO GRAMS

Ounces	*Grams*							
	1 lb.	2 lb.	3 lb.	4 lb.	5 lb.	6 lb.	7 lb.	8 lb.
0	454	907	1361	1814	2268	2722	3175	3629
1	482	936	1389	1843	2296	2750	3204	3657
2	510	964	1418	1871	2325	2778	3232	3686
3	539	992	1446	1899	2353	2807	3260	3714
4	567	1021	1474	1928	2381	2835	3289	3742
5	595	1049	1503	1956	2410	2863	3317	3771
6	624	1077	1531	1985	2438	2892	3345	3799
7	652	1106	1559	2013	2466	2920	3374	3827
8	680	1134	1588	2041	2495	2948	3402	3856
9	709	1162	1616	2070	2523	2977	3430	3884
10	737	1191	1644	2098	2552	3005	3459	3912
11	765	1219	1673	2126	2580	3033	3487	3941
12	794	1247	1701	2155	2608	3062	3515	3969
13	822	1276	1729	2183	2637	3090	3544	3997
14	851	1304	1758	2211	2665	3119	3572	4026
15	879	1332	1786	2240	2693	3147	3600	4054

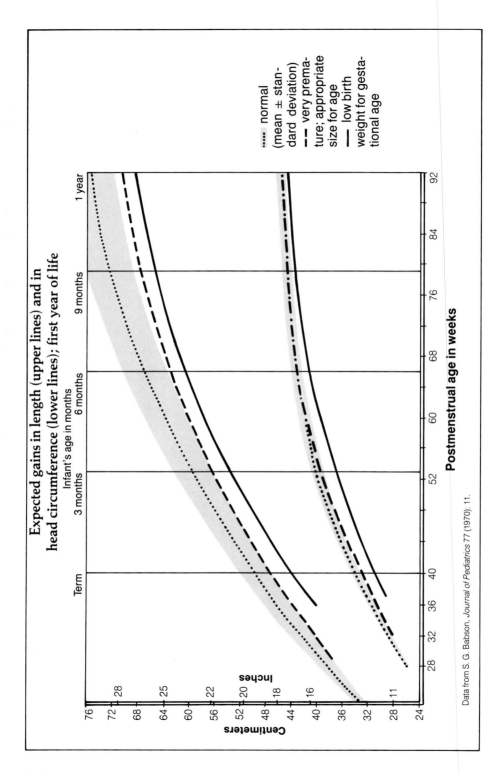

Expected gains in length (upper lines) and in head circumference (lower lines); first year of life

Data from S. G. Babson, *Journal of Pediatrics 77* (1970): 11.

legend:
- ▪▪▪ normal (mean ± standard deviation)
- – – very premature; appropriate size for age
- —— low birth weight for gestational age

Postmenstrual age in weeks

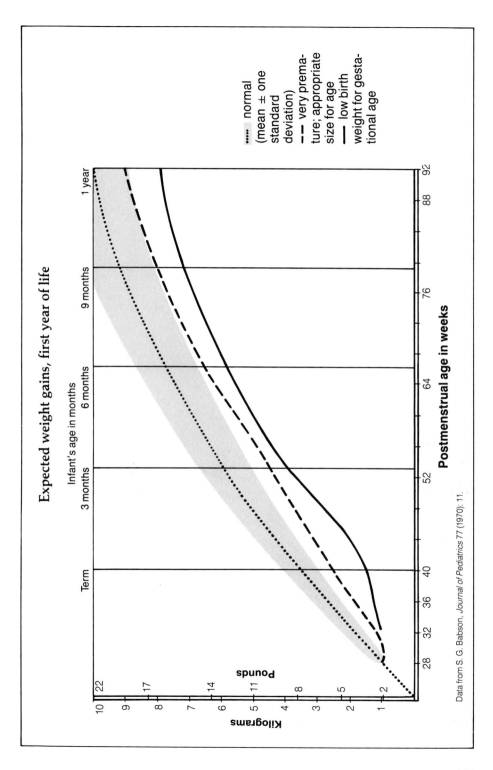

Expected weight gains, first year of life

normal (mean ± one standard deviation)

-- very premature; appropriate size for age

— low birth weight for gestational age

Infant's age in months

Term   3 months   6 months   9 months   1 year

Kilograms
10
9
8
7
6
5
4
3
2
1

Pounds
22
17
14
11
8
5
2

Postmenstrual age in weeks
28 32 36 40 52 64 76 88 92

Data from S. G. Babson, *Journal of Pediatrics* 77 (1970): 11.

Selected References

Avery, G. *Neonatology*. 2d ed. Philadelphia, J. B. Lippincott, 1981.

Avery, M. E., B. D. Fletcher, and R. G. Williams. *The Lung and Its Disorders in the Newborn Infant*. 4th ed. Philadelphia: W. B. Saunders Co., 1981.

Avery, M. E., and H. W. Taeusch, Jr. *Schaffer's Diseases of the Newborn*. 5th ed. Philadelphia: W. B. Saunders Co., 1983.

Bayley, N. *Bayley Scales of Infant Development: Birth to Two Years*. New York: Psychological Corp., 1969.

Cloherty, J. P., and A. R. Stark. *Manual of Neonatal Care*. Boston: Little, Brown and Co., 1980.

Hardy, J. B., J. S. Drage, and E. C. Jackson. *The First Year of Life*. Baltimore: Johns Hopkins University Press, 1979.

Klaus, M. H., and A. A. Fanaroff. *Care of the High-Risk Neonate*. 2d ed. Philadelphia: W. B. Saunders Co., 1979.

Rowe, R. D., R. M. Freedom, A. Mehrizi, and K. Bloom. *The Neonate with Congenital Heart Disease*. 2d ed. Philadelphia: W. B. Saunders Co., 1981.

Silverman, W. A. *Retrolental Fibroplasia: A Modern Parable*. New York: Grune Stratton, 1980.

Smith, D. W. *Recognizable Patterns of Human Malformation*. 2d ed. Philadelphia: W. B. Saunders Co., 1976.

Volpe, J. J. *Neurology of the Unborn*. Philadelphia: W. B. Saunders Co., 1981.

Index

Faierman, Dr. Alvin, 33
Fat, 45, 63, 84, 85, 108
Fathers. *See* Parents
Feeding: gavage, 87, 94–96; historical treatment of premature infants, 27–28; at home, 119; infant's responses to, 76, 92–93; after intensive care, 105, 108; in intensive care, 36, 37, 44, 45, 46, 79, 85–90; solid food, 132; vitamins in, 91, 94. *See also* Intravenous nutrition
Feelings: bonding, 39–43; long-term outlook, 136; mother and daughter, 114; mother's and feeding, 88; parents' about intensive care, 44, 46, 47, 49, 55, 66, 75, 135–136; parents' about premature birth, 17, 23, 33–34, 112; and responsibilities of baby at home, 125, 133; and transfer to Beth Israel Hospital, 105
Fetal alcohol syndrome, 20
Fetus: of lamb, 30; and preventing premature birth, 18; size of, 22; and vitamins, 91, 94
Fibroid tumors, 21
Finkelstein, Dr. Heinrich, 25
Fischer, Dr. Pamela, 48–49, 102
Folacin, 94
Folate, 94, 98
Fontanelle, 55
Formula: iron in, 91; in medical records, 98, 99; use in historical feeding, 27; vitamin C in, 94

Gastric secretions, 99
Gastrointestinal tract, 54, 67, 69, 87, 90
Gavage feeding, 87, 94–96
German measles, 52
Glucocorticoids, 60–61
Goat, 38
Growth: "catch-up," 131, 137–138; charts, 63, 150–151

Hair, 45, 79
Handling, 39, 77, 97
Hand-washing, 59
Harlow, H. F., 38–39
Harlow, M. K., 38–39
Head, 33, 35; circumference, 121, 150
Hearing, 76, 115, 119, 122
Hearing aids, 115
Heart: at discharge examination, 121; and fetal alcohol syndrome, 20; historical studies of fetal, 30; patent ductus and, 69–70, 72, 73. *See also* Heart rate
Heart operation, 69–73
Heart rate: in Apgar score, 34, 35; and apneic spells, 80–81; increase in, 70, 76; in medical records, 97, 101; monitoring in intensive care,

31, 35, 36, 37, 44, 70, 76, 80–81, 84; monitoring in transport incubator, 106
Heat shields, 57, 63
"Heel stick," 81
Height, 120, 137–138, 150
Hemoglobin, 51, 91
Hemorrhage, intraventricular, 55–56, 121
Hepatitis: infectious, 49, 52, 96; serum, 88
Hess, Dr. Julius, 25
Home: baby in, 124–133; discharge to, 119–124
Hormones, 60
Hot-water bottles, 25
Hyaline membrane disease, 28–29, 59, 60–62, 72–73, 82
Hydration, 85
Hydrocephalus, 55
Hypersegmentation, 94

Incubators: and breathing irregularities, 80; discharge from, 108, 119; and hepatitis, 96, 97; historical development of, 25, 26, 28, 29; and oxygen therapy, 64; transport, 105–107; use in intensive care, 36, 37, 44, 49, 57, 63, 76, 77, 78, 104
Indirect ophthalmoscopy, 110, 111
Indomethacin, 70, 82
Infections: control of in historical treatment, 25, 28; and death of low birth-weight infants, 23, 137; and jaundice, 51, 52, 53–54; maternal and premature birth, 21; and maturation, 138; milk as protection from, 87, 88; pregnancy and, 33; preventions of, 59; and umbilical catheters, 67, 68
Infectious hepatitis, 49, 52
Inferior vena cava, 53, 67
Infusion pump, 36, 90
Intensive care. *See* Neonatal intensive care
Intermittent mechanical ventilation (IMV), 62
Intestines, 47, 54, 85
Intrauterine environment, 51
Intrauterine growth retardation, 137, 138
Intravenous alimentation. *See* Intravenous nutrition
Intravenous fluids: in intensive care, 35, 40, 44, 57; and jaundice treatment, 53–54; in medical records, 97, 101; and umbilical catheters, 67. *See also* Intravenous nutrition
Intravenous nutrition, 27; in intensive care, 36, 37, 44, 45, 84, 85; withdrawal from, 82, 87, 88, 90, 105. *See also* Feeding; Intravenous fluids
Intraventricular hemorrhage (IVH), 55–56, 121
Iron, 91

Sugar, 28, 90, 98
Surfactant, 60, 61, 62
Survival of premature infants, 18, 23–31, 136–137
Swaddling, 43, 76

Tarnier, Dr. Etienne, 26, 27
Teeth, 87
Temporal artery, 64, 68
Temperature, nursery, 25–26. *See also* Body temperature
Theophylline, 81, 82
Thorax, 66
Tocopherol, 91
Trachea, 34, 37, 72
Transcutaneous oxygen monitor, 66
Transport incubator, 105–107
Triplets, 21
Tubs, 25, 79
Tubes: feeding, 36, 79, 87, 94; and first days in intensive care, 35, 37; in heel stick test, 81; historical use in feeding, 27; and oxygen therapy, 64; resuscitation, 34; spinal taps, 55; ventilator, 62, 65, 67
Twins, 21
Tyrosine, 94

Ultrasound: and ductus arteriosus, 70; and fetal size, 22; and heart problems, 68; and ventricular size, 55
Umbilical artery, 64, 67
Umbilical catheters, 67–69
Umbilical cord, 30, 69
Umbilical vein, 53, 67
Urinary tract disease, 21
Urine, 21, 97, 98
Uterus, 18, 21, 30, 33, 46, 60

Vaginal discharge, 18
Veins: and exchange transfusion, 53; and umbilical catheters, 67–68, 69; and intravenous nutrition, 36, 37, 87, 90
Ventilation. *See* Respiration
Ventilators. *See* Respirators
Ventricles, cerebral, 55, 56, 121
Vital signs, 44, 97, 101
Vitamin B, 94
Vitamin C, 94
Vitamin D, 91
Vitamin E, 91, 98
Vitamins, 91, 94, 98

Water, 53, 85
Water bed, 80, 82
Weber, Adrienne: at Beth Israel Hospital, 17, 108–118; birth of, 17, 33–34; body temperature, 63, 102, 103; breathing irregularities, 80, 81, 82; CAT scan and, 55, 56; cost of care for, 138, 139; and feeding, 87–90, 92–93, 95–96; first days in intensive care, 35, 37, 44–49; getting ready to go home, 119–123; growth charts of, 63; at home, 125–135; and hyaline membrane disease, 62, 82; and jaundice, 36, 49, 50, 54; length of, 104; medical record of, 98, 99, 101; named, 38; and oxygen therapy, 65; parents' bonding with, 39, 40, 41; parents' responses to, 34–35, 41–43, 75; patent ductus and, 70, 82; respiration of, 59, 82; responses to intensive care, 75, 77–79, 83–84; and retrolental fibroplasia, 110, 111; transfer to Beth Israel Hospital, 105–108; transfer to Children's Hospital Medical Center, 17, 34, 39, 41; ultrasound test, 68; and umbilical catheters, 67; vitamins for, 91; weight measurements of, 63, 85, 86, 104
Weber, Franci: and Adrienne at Beth Israel Hospital, 111, 112, 114; with Adrienne in intensive care, 75, 78–79, 80, 83; and Adrienne's birth, 32–35; and Adrienne's first days of intensive care, 44, 46–47, 49, 54, 55; and Adrienne's transfer to Beth Israel Hospital, 105; and baby at home, 119, 124–133; and bonding, 39, 40, 41, 42, 43; curiosity about intensive care, 57, 59; and dexamethasone, 33, 61; and feeding Adrienne, 46, 79, 85, 87–89, 92–93, 96, 119; feelings about premature infant, 135–136; pregnancy of, 32
Weber, Mark: and Adrienne at Beth Israel Hospital, 111, 112, 113; and Adrienne at home, 124–127, 133; with Adrienne in intensive care, 78, 80, 84, 92; and Adrienne's first days in intensive care, 44, 46, 49, 54, 55; and Adrienne's transfer to Beth Israel Hospital, 105; background, 32; and bonding, 39, 40, 41–42, 43; curiosity about intensive care, 57, 59; feelings about premature infant, 135–136
Weight, infant: birth and historical treatment, 23–24, 27–28; and feeding, 85, 86; and going home, 119, 120; in growth charts, 63, 151; hearing loss and low birth weight, 115; and incubator vs. crib, 108; and long-term outlook, 136–138; and maturation, 131, 133; in medical records, 97, 98, 104; and multiple

births, 21–22; and premature birth, 17–18, 19–20; and retrolental fibroplasia, 110

Wet nursing, 88
Wheezing, 19, 62
White blood cells, 33, 94
Windpipe. *See* Trachea

X-ray: and CAT scan, 55–56; first days in intensive care, 46; and patent ductus, 70, 71, 72–73

Ylppo, Arvo, 25